Praise for *100 Questions & Answers About Breast Cancer Sensuality, Sexuality, and Intimacy*

"Drs. Michael Krychman, Susan Kellogg Spadt, and Sandra Finestone have brought together their collective wisdom and expertise to write an outstanding book about sexual and relational well-being for breast cancer survivors and their loved ones. They provide practical tips and accessible resources for maintaining sexual wellness throughout treatment and beyond. This comprehensive and compassionate guide is a 'must read' for breast cancer survivors, their partners, and the healthcare professionals who treat them."

Sabitha Pillai-Friedman, PhD, LCSW, CST
Couple Therapist and AASECT-Certified Sex Therapist
Director of Supervisors, Jefferson/Council for Relationships
Couple and Family Therapy Program

"A breast cancer diagnosis can unravel your world. Maintaining or regaining intimacy and your sexuality after the treatment of cancer should not be a chore. *100 Questions & Answers About Breast Cancer Sensuality, Sexuality, and Intimacy* is the resource every woman needs to not just survive the treatment of her cancer but to thrive in her interpersonal relationships. This is a 'must read' for every woman diagnosed with breast cancer and her doctors!"

Beth Baughman DuPree, MD, FACS
Chairman of the American Society of Breast Surgeons Board of Advocates
Author of The Healing Consciousness: A Doctor's Journey to Healing

"In just 100 answers, the authors of this book address many of the issues facing women with breast cancer. From decisions about surgery to hormones and sex toys, the authors address the many questions that these women have thought—or may need to think about."

Anne Katz, RN, PhD
Author of Breaking the Silence on Cancer and Sexuality *and* Women Cancer Sex

"Dr. Michael Krychman and his colleagues have done it again with another great book addressing key questions and answers about life after breast cancer. Many doctors often don't have the time or the expertise to discuss sexuality, intimacy, and relationships after treatment of breast cancer. Michael Krychman, Susan Kellogg Spadt, and Sandy Finestone understand that sexuality after breast cancer is important and needs to be addressed. This fabulous book provides clear, easy-to-understand solutions for the reader who is often too embarrassed to raise these concerns with their own doctor. It is an excellent book not only for patients but also doctors and nurses who care for women after treatment of breast cancer."

John Boyages, MD
Director, Westmead Breast Cancer Institute
Sydney Australia
Author of Breast Cancer: Taking Control
www.breastcancertakingcontrol.com

"This is a book filled with wisdom, compassion, and wise counsel from a phenomenal team of authors. I believe that every woman with breast cancer and her partner who reads this book will find hope and useful advice."

Dr. Stephanie Buehler
Psychologist and Sex Therapist
Director, The Buehler Institute

"This book is reminiscent of the necessary supportive companion through any woman's struggle and journey with breast cancer. By answering 100 of the most common sexual health-related questions encountered by healthcare providers working with cancer survivors, Dr. Krychman, Dr. Kellogg Spadt, and Ms. Finestone offer one of the most comprehensive and accessible guides to understanding, learning, and growing from sexual struggles that women with breast cancer experience. This book is equally valuable to the healthcare provider with its evidence-based suggestions and rich clinical examples."

Dr. Lori Brotto, PhD, R Psych
Assistant Professor
University of British Columbia

"Breast cancer (BC), today, is more of a chronic than a fatal disease for the majority of affected women. This makes the quality of life of BC survivors a critical and yet neglected issue, when sexuality and intimacy are concerned. Indeed, many studies indicate that couples' *emotional intimacy* may be reinforced by the sharing of solidarity the couple has when facing BC diagnosis and treatment, while *physical intimacy* and *physical satisfaction* appear to be definitely worsened, mostly because of biological factors usually overlooked in the clinical management of breast cancer patients.

Women are left alone, sexuality being a persistent taboo among oncologic professionals, with a few exceptions. Think of it. The underlying message is just one: be happy that you are alive. This cannot be accepted anymore.

Being back to a meaningful and fulfilling life, after a challenging diagnostic and therapeutic time, means that the happiness of a sexually happy body cannot be neglected anymore as a marginal issue. Michael Krychman, Susan Kellogg Spadt, and Sandy Finestones' book is, therefore, timely and much needed; it goes to the heart of what intimacy and sexuality mean in *real life* for BC survivors and their partners.

It will certainly be precious for women. My heartfelt wish is that it will be read and meditated upon by all healthcare professionals who work with BC survivors, to break the 'collusion of silence' about sexuality. The woman is too scared or afraid or shy to ask, the professional too busy to think of it. And yet, it is very difficult to provide an effective intervention if there is no mention of a problem!

This is the best gift we can give to every woman who has gone through the dramatic months of breast cancer diagnosis and treatments: the beauty of feeling sensual and sexual, aroused and orgasmic, physically and emotionally happy again, with the partner she loves."

Alessandra Graziottin, MD
Specialist in Gynecology, Oncology and Sexual Medicine
Director, Center of Gynecology and Medical Sexology
H. San Raffaele Resnati,

"With one in seven American women being affected by breast cancer, it is about time someone finally tackled the intimacy issues that plague our survivors. The authors have demystified critical, yet often unspoken, concerns of our patients. They have created a vehicle to assist women in opening discussion and with the ultimate goal of facilitating treatment for sexual concerns that, if left unaddressed, have the potential to devastate the lives that they have fought so hard to keep."

Alison Amsterdam, MD, FACP
Assistant Professor, Mount Sinai School of Medicine

"Drs. Michael Krychman and Susan Kellogg Spadt provide an invaluable and inspirational resource for women who are on the journey through breast cancer diagnosis and beyond. This book is a practical guide for breast cancer survivors who are on the journey to recapturing intimacy and well-being, providing guidance for some of the most commonly asked questions that face cancer survivors."

Arti Hurria, MD
Associate Professor of Medicine
Director, Cancer and Aging Research Program
Breast Cancer Oncologist, City of Hope Cancer Center

"In to the field of breast cancer and cancer survivorship comes a much needed resource for women and their partners. In writing *100 Questions & Answers About Breast Cancer Sensuality, Sexuality, and Intimacy*, Drs. Krychman and Kellogg Spadt, alongside Ms. Finestone, have provided an educated, reasoned, and balanced resource for this community of women, one that constitutes the largest group of cancer survivors in the United States. This book is a testament to how breast cancer impacts more than just the patient. Breast cancer touches her partner, and affects, and indeed challenges, relationships. I hope that providers will see this as a resource for their own understanding on how to address and counsel patients whose partner relations have been affected by breast cancer. I applaud the authors on providing this timely resource. I am certain it will become a must-have for every survivorship center in the United States and worldwide."

Don S. Dizon, MD
Director, Medical Oncology and Integrative Care
Director, The Center for Sexuality, Intimacy, and Fertility
The Program in Women's Oncology at Women & Infants' Hospital
Assistant Professor, The Warren Alpert Medical School of Brown University

"Dr. Krychman, Dr. Kellogg Spadt, and Ms. Finestone have successfully integrated three very different perspectives on cancer and sexual medicine, the result of which is this user-friendly book to help women traverse the sexual problems that accompany cancer. They effectively synthesize a vast amount of information about the complexities of women's sexuality and provide a thorough review of potential problems and treatment options including psychotherapy, physical therapy, pharmacotherapy, and herbal therapy. For cancer survivors and their lovers, this book will support and guide them."

Sheryl A. Kingsberg, PhD
Chief of the Division of Behavioral Medicine
Department of Obstetrics & Gynecology
University Hospitals of Cleveland Case Medical Center
Professor of Reproductive Biology and Psychiatry
Case Western Reserve University
President of The International Society for the Study of Women's Sexual Health

"*100 Questions & Answers About Breast Cancer Sensuality, Sexuality, and Intimacy* is a must read for patients and their partners facing a breast cancer diagnosis.

As an organization that hears from tens of thousands of breast cancer patients seeking information and emotional support, this book is a great tool for before, during, and after treatment.

No subject is off limits and ideas and facts are clearly explained to help patients and their partners find their new 'normal' and even enhance intimacy and quality of life."

The YourShoes Peer Counselors
Breast Cancer Network of Strength

"This book provides much needed attention and information to help women re-discovering or maintain intimacy after a diagnosis of breast cancer."

Ann H. Partridge, MD, MPH
Dana-Farber Cancer Institute

"'Breast cancer' is a diagnosis that no woman wants to hear. She will worry about her doctors, her treatment decisions, side effects, disease recurrence, and yes, her very survival. But even beyond physical discomforts and survival, a breast is not simply an anatomic organ, like a colon or a thyroid. Although physicians are necessarily focused on curing or slowing malignant disease, they need to acknowledge that for many women and their partners, breasts are symbolically and even functionally important. Breasts are inextricably bound to a woman's self image, to motherhood and nurturing, to attractiveness and sexuality...

Fortunately, most breast cancers today are eminently treatable and women will have many years after diagnosis to grapple with evolving issues of self image and sexuality. A new book on intimacy and sexuality after a breast cancer diagnosis by Michael Krychman, Sandra Finestone, and Susan Kellogg Spadt, is a refreshing addition to the literature. The authors help women with breast cancer and their partners—and, hopefully, the professionals who treat and care for them—face these issues frankly, with advice, with information, and always with love and hope."

Margie Miller
Group Scientific Director, Oncology
Medscape

"As a former oncology nurse who now practices Eastern medicine including acupuncture and herbal therapy, I am always looking for resources that can aid my breast cancer patients in taking a more active role in their healing. An area that is commonly overlooked by both patient and practitioner at the outset of cancer treatment is what effect the illness and subsequent treatment may have on sexual health and vitality. This wonderful book is a very straight forward, no-nonsense approach to this often sensitive and complicated subject. I applaud the authors, particularly Dr. Michael Krychman, for their dedication to the sexual health of women with cancer."

Pamela Jacobson, LAc, Dipl OM
The Healing Sanctuary

"We are comfortable talking about breast cancer today—women freely share their stories about how they were diagnosed, how they felt, what they did—with each other, in groups, even in the media. But the sensitive and private topics of intimacy and sexuality are often not comfortable topics of conversation—between patients and healthcare providers or between couples. This book will help start those conversations and serve as a guide to answers to questions that need to be discussed."

Susan Brown, RN
Director of Education
Susan G. Komen for the Cure

"Sexuality/intimacy and cancer diagnosis/treatment are words that are not often seen together. Each one of these words evoke various emotions in people living with a cancer diagnosis. Any discussion regarding sexuality and all its ramifications will be amazingly important to anyone past and present who has ever received that diagnosis. Having a book such as this helps educate an individual to understand feelings that are so often not discussed or pushed aside. It is a real gift."

Sue Winn, RN
Patient Navigator

100 Questions & Answers About Breast Cancer Sensuality, Sexuality, and Intimacy

Michael L. Krychman, MD

Medical Director Sexual Medicine
Hoag Memorial Hospital
Newport Beach, CA

Susan Kellogg Spadt, PhD, CRNP

Co-Director, The Pelvic & Sexual Health Institute of Philadelphia
Director of Sexual Medicine
Philadelphia, PA

with

Sandra Finestone, PsyD

Executive Director
Hope and Wellness Center
Costa Mesa, CA

JONES & BARTLETT
LEARNING

World Headquarters
Jones & Bartlett Learning
40 Tall Pine Drive
Sudbury, MA 01776
978-443-5000
info@jblearning.com
www.jblearning.com

Jones & Bartlett Learning
Canada
6339 Ormindale Way
Mississauga, Ontario L5V 1J2
Canada

Jones & Bartlett Learning
International
Barb House, Barb Mews
London W6 7PA
United Kingdom

Jones & Bartlett Learning books and products are available through most bookstores and online booksellers. To contact Jones & Bartlett Learning directly, call 800-832-0034, fax 978-443-8000, or visit our website, www.jblearning.com.

Substantial discounts on bulk quantities of Jones & Bartlett Learning publications are available to corporations, professional associations, and other qualified organizations. For details and specific discount information, contact the special sales department at Jones & Bartlett Learning via the above contact information or send an email to specialsales@jblearning.com.

The authors, editor, and publisher have made every effort to provide accurate information. However, they are not responsible for errors, omissions, or for any outcomes related to the use of the contents of this book and take no responsibility for the use of the products and procedures described. Treatments and side effects described in this book may not be applicable to all people; likewise, some people may require a dose or experience a side effect that is not described herein. Drugs and medical devices are discussed that may have limited availability controlled by the Food and Drug Administration (FDA) for use only in a research study or clinical trial. Research, clinical practice, and government regulations often change the accepted standard in this field. When consideration is being given to use of any drug in the clinical setting, the healthcare provider or reader is responsible for determining FDA status of the drug, reading the package insert, and reviewing prescribing information for the most up-to-date recommendations on dose, precautions, and contraindications, and determining the appropriate usage for the product. This is especially important in the case of drugs that are new or seldom used.

Production Credits
Executive Publisher: Christopher Davis
Editorial Assistant: Sara Cameron
Production Director: Amy Rose
Production Editor: Daniel Stone
Senior Marketing Manager: Barb Bartoszek

Manufacturing and Inventory Control Supervisor:
  Amy Bacus
Composition: Spoke & Wheel
Printing and Binding: Malloy, Inc.

Cover Credits
Cover Design: Carolyn Downer
Cover Images: Top Photo: © Monkey Business Images/ShutterStock, Inc.; Bottom Left Photo: © Yuri Arcurs/ShutterStock, Inc.; and Bottom Right Photo: © Stephen Coburn/ShutterStock, Inc.
Cover Printing: Malloy, Inc.

Library of Congress Cataloging-in-Publication Data
Krychman, Michael L.
100 questions & answers about breast cancer sensuality, sexuality, and intimacy / Michael L. Krychman, Susan Kellogg Spadt, Sandra Finestone.
    p. cm.
Includes index.
ISBN 978-0-7637-7909-2
1. Breast Cancer—Popular works. 2. Cancer in women—Miscellanea. I. Kellogg Spadt, Susan. II. Finestone, Sandra. III. Title. IV. Title: One hundred questions and answers about breast cancer sensuality, sexuality, and intimacy.
RC281.W65K78 2011
616.99'449—dc22
                                                                                    2010011842
6048

Printed in the United States of America
14 13 12 11 10   10 9 8 7 6 5 4 3 2 1

Michael L. Krychman, MD

I would like to thank Chris Davis and his team at Jones & Bartlett Learning for believing in this book and understanding the importance of sexual health and wellness.

To my parents who have taught me, in their own special way, that hard work, dedication, and perseverance will always guide you to success. To Susan, my co-author and colleague, you have shown me unconditional friendship and wisdom that has helped me in many ways. A special thank you to Frances Schultz for her friendship, literary support, and good humor.

To my incredible children, Julianna and Russell, you are a source of joy, love, and wonderment. I have been blessed with both of you! Thank you for allowing me to be your papa! I must also thank the love of my life, for the supportive and loving commitment to our family.

My life has been touched by strong women who have faced breast cancer—to my grandmother Rose, Tutu Kendall, and Aunt Ordie—all of you have lived and died graciously and did not let breast cancer slow you down. But especially to all the women who face cancer with pride and courage, this book is dedicated to you and your families—I can hope that with this book you may rekindle and reaffirm your relationships.

As a scientist I can speak about proteins, risk factors, and other possible medical explanations for cancer, but as a dedicated healthcare professional, I know that it is not purely the biological but also the connections to others, perhaps the compassionate words of a caring doctor, the gentle touch from a nurse, or the even random kind words from a stranger that will help women survive and thrive during the cancer experience. It is my hope that this book helps those in need and allows them to create a new intimate connectedness that will nurture, love, and provide strength.

Susan Kellogg Spadt, PhD, CRNP

My heartfelt thanks to my two esteemed collaborators on this book: Dr. Michael Krychman, an accomplished medical sexologist, my colleague, and dear friend. You are the person who introduced me to the natural relationship between sexual medicine and survivorship medicine and who continually inspires me to give 200% to my patients, my family, my friends, my writing, and my career; and Sandra Finestone, who, although we have never met face to face, has inspired me through passionate and committed writing about survivorship and sexual wellness for women.

My deepest appreciation to my wonderful and ever-supportive family. To my husband, Kirk, you have always been my biggest supporter, my inspiration, and true companion. You tirelessly "held down the fort" while I wrote and researched...I love you and my life with you! To my beautiful children, Seton and Shannon, who have matured into successful and compassionate young adults in their own right, seemingly unscathed by having a mom who is a medical sexologist (but thanks, for the times you endured any temporary embarrassment or discomfort during childhood, as a result of my profession). May you be equally passionate about your chosen fields and never compromise your ideals or standards. Excellence is within your reach!

My thanks to my amazing 90-year-old mother, who is healthy and vital in so many ways. You (along with my dear departed father) are the embodiment of the true spirit of survivorship and sexual wellness and you continue to be an inspiration for my career, my family life, and my wonderful marriage.

To my supportive associates and dear friends at the Pelvic and Sexual Health Institute of Philadelphia; Medical Director and business partner, Dr. Kristene Whitmore; and colleagues Amy Rejba Hoffman and Jennifer Yonaitis Fariello: You have witnessed and supported my interest in sexuality and survivorship and continue to provide excellent care to the patients that we serve.

Last, to the astounding women who have survived the cancer experience and who cared enough about themselves and their partners to seek consultation with me for the enrichment of their sexual lives...you have shared so much of yourselves...your experiences and your challenges. You have been the primary inspiration for me to incorporate the survivorship philosophy into my clinical practice and to coauthor this book. Thank you!

Sandra Finestone, PsyD

I dedicate this book to all the incredible women who have shared their lives, their pain, their fears, and their frustrations with me, and to my children, grandchildren, and sister who supported me in my efforts to dedicate myself to caring for these women and their families.

But it is to my husband I owe the greatest debt. He believed in me when I did not believe in myself and made me see that all things are possible if you have the right person beside you to share your dreams.

Breast cancer seems ubiquitous. Most of us have yet to meet any person professionally or personally whose life has not been touched by breast cancer. These words are common: "I know someone who was just diagnosed with breast cancer." The stories can be heartwarming (e.g., the 40-year-old workaholic who reprioritizes her life after her diagnosis to slow down by spending more time meditating, eating well, playing with her kids, and making love with her husband) and others devastating (e.g., the 52-year-old woman whose husband drops her off at the bus station so that she can go to her radiation appointment alone while he leaves for a liaison with his young mistress). Breast cancer clearly affects a woman, her family network, her sexual function, and intimacy. The diagnosis of cancer can pull strong, loving couples together or tear them apart. It can destroy their intimate bond or rekindle a previously fading sexual fire. Cancer appears almost mystical in its ability to transform relationships, both good and bad, positive and negative.

This book is written in the hopes that the intimate lives of its readers will be rekindled, rather than devastated, by the experience of breast cancer. We, the authors, are neither naïve nor unrealistic. We realize the difficulty of the cancer journey, but we are also privileged to witness the "light at the end of the tunnel" (e.g., reestablishment of sexual wellness) for our patients every day. We hope to share with you some of what our patients have taught us.

PART ONE

The Basics

What is sexual health and vitality?

Does every breast cancer survivor experience changes in her sexual health?

What aspects of sexual response (e.g., desire, arousal, orgasm, and sexual comfort) might change after breast cancer treatment?

More . . .

1. What is sexual health and vitality?

This book discusses sexual health and vitality for breast **cancer** survivors. Although one author is a medical doctor, one a nurse practitioner, and the third a social worker, all are professional sexologists and work each day with inspiring breast cancer survivors. We speak with one voice as we discuss the difficult sexual challenges that individuals and couples face after cancer, as well as the transformative power that reestablishing sexual health can have for a woman and her partner.

What is sexual health? How do I know whether I am sexually vital? Is it possible to regain the level of sexual wellness that I had before my diagnosis and treatment? For every couple, sexual health and vitality are different and unique (e.g., how you feel as a sexual person, how you "connect" with your partner, or the attitudes you cherish toward your sexual activity).

Recently, the National Women's Health Resource Center, in cooperation with the Association of Reproductive Health Professionals and Boehringer-Ingelheim Pharmaceuticals, conducted a nationally representative survey of 1,200 women (ages 18–50 years) in the United States to look at female sexual health. The survey found that 81% of women believe that sexual health is important for overall health but that 70% had experienced some difficulty (unfortunately, only 18% had consulted with a healthcare provider). Women ranked a healthy sex life higher in importance than career satisfaction, home ownership, travel, and social life. When asked about their sexual health, women conceptualize healthy sexuality differently, especially in terms of *quantity* (e.g., having **intercourse** two to three times per week or three to four times per month). Surprisingly, nearly 80% of the women

Cancer

A disease characterized by uncontrolled cell growth that ultimately causes destruction of normal healthy tissue.

Intercourse

Sexual contact usually involving coitus or penile vaginal penetration.

who participated agreed about *quality*. They felt that a woman was truly healthy when she

1. Had a satisfying sex life.
2. Had a good relationship with her partner.
3. Experienced some level of sexual satisfaction.

This book addresses all of the areas of sexual health, citing examples from our clinical practices and from the sexual health literature.

2. Does every breast cancer survivor experience changes in her sexual health?

The American Cancer Society estimates that approximately 90% of breast cancer survivors experience some alteration in their **sexuality**. This could be on the outside (e.g., how a woman's body looks or how her genitals, **vagina**, **vulva**, or **clitoris** may react to stimulation) or on the inside (e.g., how a woman feels about herself, her level of sexual desire, and/or her attitudes about being with her partner). Despite this high percentage, most women are able to redefine "adequate and satisfying" sexual activity and reclaim a sense of normalcy of physical intimacy.

3. What aspects of sexual response (e.g., desire, arousal, orgasm, and sexual comfort) might change after breast cancer treatment?

Any or all aspects of sexual response might change after breast cancer treatment. The categories of sexual disorders include

The American Cancer Society estimates that approximately 90% of breast cancer survivors experience some alteration in their sexuality.

THE BASICS

Sexuality
The feelings, behaviors, and identities associated with sex.

Vagina
The part of the female genital tract that connects the uterus to the external vulva. It is 8 to 10 cm in length.

Vulva
The external genital organs of the female, including the labia majora, labia minora, clitoris, and vestibule of the vagina.

Clitoris
The erectile organ in women whose external portion is located at the junction of the labia minora just in front of the vestibule.

3

- Desire—motivation to engage in sexual activity or thoughts/fantasies about sexual intimacy.
- Arousal—mental and physical excitability in response to sexual stimulation. How does your vagina or vulva feel when stimulated? Some may experience a tingling or fullness in the pelvic region.
- **Orgasm**—a diminished, delayed, or absent peak in the intensity of sexual excitement.
- Sexual pain—genital and/or pelvic pain that occurs before, during, or after sexual activity. Pain may be on the inside (with vaginal pain) or the outside. Vulvar dryness may also cause sexual pain in some cancer patients, causing tenderness on penetration.

Approximately 10% to 70% of breast cancer survivors report that they struggle with **libido**. This is common when dealing with a serious medical health issue, as high levels of stress and changes in family and relationship dynamics may exist.

Physical discomfort, from mild irritation to severe sexual pain, is common in breast cancer survivors. Because of lowered **estrogen** levels in the body (from many cancer treatments), women may find that sexual stimulation no longer produces high levels of vaginal wetness and arousal. In addition, regardless of how "turned on" she feels before and during intercourse, a woman's genitals might feel dry and raw, and she might experience pain with penetration and thrusting movements, making it much harder to reach an orgasm.

These very predictable changes require a little creativity for a woman and her partner. Sexually healthy survivors are able to explain to their partners that changes in **lubrication** needs and sexual discomfort are expected

Orgasm

The intense pleasurable sensation at the peak of sexual activity or sexual climax usually associated with spasmodic contraction of the pelvic floor muscles. It is often associated with ejaculation, especially in men.

Libido

Sexual interest or desire.

Estrogen

A steroid hormone produced mainly in the ovaries; the primary female sexual hormone.

Lubrication

The natural appearance of slippery secretions in the vagina during sexual arousal or the use of artificial lubricants to facilitate sexual activity or intercourse.

results from cancer treatments. Together, women and their partners can choose suitable vaginal moisturizers and vulvar lubricants and apply them before and during sex to make intercourse (see Question 75).

4. From a sexual health perspective, which couples adjust well and which do not after breast cancer and why?

One of the most important predictors of sexual vitality *after* breast cancer is sexual vitality *before* breast cancer. Couples who were able to "handle" life events such as child rearing, work or financial stressors, moves, and illnesses are typically able to adjust their sexual styles to accommodate for the changes associated with breast cancer; however, even if a woman's sexual life was *not* optimal before breast cancer, she is not destined for failure. By mobilizing the myriad of available healthcare and other support services (e.g., reading this book with a partner), women can secure future physical intimacy and sexual vitality.

For success in coping with sexual changes, women and their partners must be flexible and keep a sense of openness in the relationship. Although sex might be different in some ways, change does not mean inferior—just different. Survivors who are most successful at reclaiming their sexual vitality are able to maintain a strong sense of "sexual self-esteem." Doing so, however, may require exploring new methods of pleasuring oneself or a partner, taking extra time to "prepare" for sex (with lubricants, moisturizers, creams, and arousal aids), trying new sexual positions, and limiting the amount of time that a **penis** or self-stimulator/vibrator is inside the vagina. These changes, although minor, can facilitate sexual communication and a healthy overall adaptation after breast cancer.

Penis

The erectile, sexually erotically sensitive organ in males. The penis serves a sexual function and also mediates the voiding of urine.

THE BASICS

5. *Do most breast cancer survivors need help in dealing with sexual changes after breast cancer?*

Each woman reacts differently to the sexual changes that accompany breast cancer diagnosis, treatment, and survivorship.

Each woman reacts differently to the sexual changes that accompany breast cancer diagnosis, treatment, and survivorship. Many benefit from the help that sexual medicine specialists, counselors, and/or therapists offer (in addition to the expert advice that they receive from their primary healthcare providers and oncologists). The specialist will likely have encountered the same issue when working with other survivors. He or she will be aware of the fastest, safest, and most successful strategies to address changes in sexual desire, vaginal dryness, physical discomfort during sex, or orgasm difficulties.

Magnolia Myrick:

I was in my 40s when the diagnosis came, single, not menopausal, sexually active in theory, if not in practice, at that moment.

If you're single, first you worry about the dating, and then you worry about the sex. I was seriously worried about losing my sex drive and/or my sex appeal. The cancer's bad enough, but I've got to lose my "mojo" too? Please. I was totally unprepared for this, and my healthcare providers didn't bring it up until I asked. Perhaps they, understandably, didn't want to burden a patient with more not so great news than she was already dealing with. I'm going to go into menopause because of chemotherapy? A doctor didn't tell me that—a friend did. That's a pretty big piece of information.

So, menopause...a common symptom is vaginal dryness, which can cause pain during intercourse. After several months of abstinence, I became sexually active again about halfway through the 4-month chemo treatment. Ouch! I had no idea the vagina would not only be drier but would lose some of its elasticity. (I know, but I had enough to think about already.) The good news is that it doesn't have to stay that way. Apart from the lubricants and moisturizers, you can also use vaginal dilators and good old-fashioned dildos and vibrators to keep yourself in sexual shape. (The Internet is full of sources for these things—it's a riot!) My gynecologist, however, ordered the dilators.

I was mortified to broach the sexuality subject with a health-care provider, let alone my oncologist, but I was even more mortified at the prospect of a crummy sex life and refused to accept it. "Use it or lose it," my doctor said, and keep those "neural pathways" open and flowing. In other words, keep having orgasms, self-induced or otherwise. Now that's my kind of prescription.

If your doctor is less than enthusiastic about discussing this and offering practical (if embarrassing) advice, then ask to be referred to someone who is. The specialists—physicians, therapists, or counselors—tend to talk about sex very matter-of-factly, like it was the laundry or something, and it makes you able to discuss it matter-of-factly also (almost!).

6. What type of healthcare professional is trained to help women with these issues?

Marriage and family therapists focus on the psychological dynamics of couple relationships and the broad array of sexual challenges that many couples face. Sex therapists, marriage and family therapists, psychologists, and/or social workers have had specific training about sexuality and can address complex issues in an efficient manner. To assure quality in a sexual health provider, look for certification of the American Association of Sex Educators

Counselors and Therapists, which is the certifying body for sexual health specialists. Certification, a voluntary activity, is often a lengthy process and requires evidence of specialized training, hours of patient contact, and verification of competency in the field of sexual health by other sexual health specialists. Also, sexual counselors and sexual therapists, as well as medical doctors and nurse providers, specialize in the diagnosis and treatment of sexual complaints from breast cancer patients. A good reference may be the International Society for the Study of Women's Sexual Health, as well as American Cancer Society. The International Society of Sexual Medicine may also be helpful when you are trying to locate a healthcare provider who is sensitive to sexual health, wellness, and cancer care.

7. What is sexual medicine?

Sexual medicine embraces the study, diagnosis, and treatment of sexual health concerns of women and men. Specialists are usually doctors or nurse practitioners who have a background in family medicine, obstetrics and gynecology, or urology; they have attended specific sexual health-related academic programs, training courses, or preceptorships. Although sexual medicine is not now a standardized medical education path, it is gaining wide acceptance throughout the United States and Europe (see Question 6). Specialists, often called medical sexologists, focus on sexual concerns through a comprehensive sexual history, a thorough physical examination, and adjuvant specialized testing. Sexual medicine specialists may treat sexual health concerns with

- Prescription medication
- Physical therapy
- Surgery

- Psychotherapy and psychosexual counseling
- Behavioral counseling
- Complementary and alternative therapies
- Any combination of these

Sexual medicine specialists are often concerned with enhancing the overall quality of the couple relationship and may see both partners during the therapeutic treatment period. Sexual medicine specialists can also be American Association of Sex Educators Counselors and Therapists-certified as sexuality educators, counselors, or therapists.

8. What is survivorship medicine?

An exciting transformation has taken place about what it means to be affected by cancer. Rather than seeing and being seen as an unfortunate "victim," individuals see and feel themselves empowered as survivors or "thrivers." A recent feature article in *Psychology Today* notes that survivorship is increasingly common, with approximately 11.4 million Americans well after treatment. Survivors are often vocal about their experiences and may feel empowered by their diagnosis and their experiences undergoing difficult, but effective, treatment strategies. Increasingly, celebrities make public disclosure of their cancer diagnosis and see spreading the word as a profound aspect of their public persona. New research on the survivorship experience suggests that when individuals with cancer emerge victorious after experiencing highly intense medical treatments, relationship stressors, and other life changes, they are more resilient and demonstrate qualities of personal strength and vitality that they never knew they had.

The survivorship philosophy is now embraced and well supported by a new movement in health care. Survivorship medicine focuses on optimizing prevention and wellness after cancer. Prevention of other diseases caused by initial cancer care is also addressed. Healthcare providers who practice this form of care are committed to cancer prevention and early detection, as well as using medications, behavior modification, exercise, diet, stress management, counseling, sex therapy, and alternative medical approaches to ensure quality of life for cancer survivors.

Survivorship medicine emphasizes living with a disease diagnosis and disease prevention rather than focusing on disease-imposed limitations or restrictions.

Survivorship medicine emphasizes living with a disease diagnosis and disease prevention rather than focusing on disease-imposed limitations or restrictions. It sees a patient as a survivor rather than as a victim and addresses complex postcancer issues such as pain management, family systems, and minimization of disability.

Magnolia Myrick:

I don't suppose you ever feel quite the same after having cancer. Even if the doctors say they've "gotten it all," the fact of it lingers. You know it happened, and you know it can happen again. Even sometime in the distant future! Not a great thing to have hanging over your head. And hanging. But you don't have to stand there under it all the time, either, now do you?

What I don't always know is how other people feel about me after having cancer. Do they see me as weak? Sickly? "Damaged goods"? Some probably do. And that's their problem. I can't remember who said, "What other people think of me is none of my business," but it's a great saying. And the truth is other people are not sitting around thinking about me all that much anyway. They might gossip about me for a few minutes, but then they'll go right back to thinking about themselves and their own problems, like they always do.

As a practical matter, I didn't tell the people I worked with about having cancer. I am a self-employed freelance writer, and I didn't want editors to avoid giving me assignments because they didn't think I was up to it. I wanted to make that decision, thank you. So I kept word of my health status to close friends and family. Now you can't always control what people know about you, but I let it be known that I wanted to be very low key about it. I didn't want it to be what my life was about. I also didn't want to exhaust myself talking about it to people I wasn't close to.

Another thing that changes after cancer is how you feel about other people, namely friends and family who may—or may not—have been a great support to you. Cancer is nothing if not a test of character, for the patient and for the patient's family and friends as well. Yes, some people will perceive you differently, or even fearfully, because you've had cancer. And while it is well and good to say they feel this way because of their own fears and insecurities, I think it is also due to a lack of character. I wouldn't necessarily end a relationship over it, but I would see it differently and value it less, frankly.

9. What information does my healthcare providers need to know to assist me with my sexual health?

Specialists in sexual health are skilled in working with survivor issues and concerns. By consulting with a specialist, issues about your innermost sexual fears or concerns that may seem "silly" can be taken seriously and addressed accordingly. Talk about your first sexual experiences, any instance of sexual abuse, sexual preferences, types and number of sexual partners, and activities in which you engage. By sharing these very personal details, a professional can help you work toward your goals and facilitate your healthy adjustment and movement through this phase of your life.

Often, a sexual healthcare provider can be an advocate for sharing sensitive topics with your partner. Most sexual health specialists are comfortable using sexually explicit terms, understand traditional and alternative sexual practices, and are trained to deal with desire discrepancy concerns, body image issues, and sexual pain. They typically focus on sexual health issues in a more comprehensive fashion than other members of your breast cancer treatment team.

10. Should I discuss sexual health issues with my oncologist(s), or should I wait until they are brought up with me?

Always bring up sexual health issues with your healthcare provider(s), even if you feel embarrassed or are unsure about which words to use. Although most oncologists, obstetrician/gynecologists, and family practice medical providers believe that sexual health is vital to an individual's overall health, they are often focused on other issues surrounding cancer diagnosis, treatment, and follow-up or may feel time constraints during their busy clinic day. They may feel that if sexual health were an issue the patient would voice a concern.

Your oncologist has likely heard similar concerns in the past and may have a list of qualified referrals for sexuality-focused psychological counseling or medical care. Asking for help may be the first step toward your sexual comfort, renewed interest, and overall satisfaction.

Magnolia Myrick:

Honey, if having cancer hasn't taught you to be proactive about your health and everything else in your life, now would be a good time to start. Nobody's going to do it for you as well as you can. Absolutely ask your healthcare provider anything. At worst, she or he doesn't know the answer and can refer you to someone who does. Not asking has far worse consequences than overcoming a little shyness. You're the one in charge here. And I promise: You will feel so good and so relieved that you did bring it up, you will wonder why on earth you hesitated in the first place.

PART TWO

Treatments

Is sexual functioning different for those who have had a mastectomy or lumpectomy?

My husband hasn't made any effort to see me naked since the surgery. Why?

I am too tired for sex. How can I decrease my fatigue level?

More . . .

11. Is sexual functioning different for those who have had a mastectomy or lumpectomy?

Mastectomy

The removal of the breast.

Lumpectomy

Removal of a small amount of tissue of the breast including the abnormal cancerous cells.

Most women with breast cancer will require some form of surgery (e.g., a **mastectomy** or a **lumpectomy**). Often, the oncological surgeon will discuss which option will offer the best chance for cure; however, you might worry about how the operative procedures may change the way your body looks. Health literature does not support the fact that women who undergo a complete mastectomy do better or worse than those who have breast-conservation surgery. After an adequate period of recovery, the two groups did not differ with respect to sexual satisfaction, orgasm, and sexual frequency. In fact, many women enjoyed the postoperative sexual response; however, women who had total breast tissue removed had less breast caressing.

Oncoplastic surgery

Surgery in which a tumor is removed by either mastectomy or lumpectomy. Immediate reconstruction is performed at the time of surgery.

Mammoplasty

Plastic surgery of the breasts; reduction—making breasts smaller; augmentation—making breasts larger.

Mammopexy

Breast lifting plastic surgical procedure.

A mastectomy or other operative changes in your breasts may affect your self-esteem and influence how you view yourself. With extensive surgical resection and radical surgery and surgical scarring, some women shift their perceptions of their bodies and femininity.

12. What is oncoplastic surgery?

In **oncoplastic surgery**, a tumor is removed and immediate reconstruction is performed to ensure satisfactory cosmetic results. Sometimes a flap of tissue with its blood supply and nerves is moved from one area of the body to another, and through delicate and careful surgical techniques, the breast is reconstructed. Sometimes oncoplastic surgery may require a reduction **mammoplasty**, or breast reduction in the unaffected breast, to ensure symmetry. Sometimes **mammopexy**, or breast lift, is also done on the unaffected breast. This helps the breasts to appear symmetrical. Sometimes nipples are removed. Multiple surgeons are often involved in this process.

Although surgeons and patients hope for excellent cosmetic results, sometimes the surgical effect is less favorable than expected. Some interventions, such as **Scarguard**, may be used to lessen the intensity and color of the scars. Sometimes nipples can be reconstructed by other tissue or permanent tattooing done in the nipple area. Sometimes prostheses may be available. If you are unhappy with the way your new breasts look or want to consider reconstructive surgery, ask your healthcare team for a plastic surgery consultation. There are new and innovative ways to help your breasts regain their vitality they once had.

Ask questions. Ask to see books with results, and ask whether your healthcare professionals have had experience with reconstructive surgery in breast cancer patients.

Scarguard

A topical skin-care product designed to be used to minimize the appearance of scars from injury and surgery.

13. Should I have reconstruction? Will it help with my sexual self-esteem?

Surgical reconstruction is a personal choice. Some women do not mind having only one breast, whereas others do. Consider your feelings about the issue before embarking on consultation after consultation; having reconstructive surgery for the wrong reasons can be harmful. Sometimes if women feel as if they are "damaged," surgery may help them recover from the anxieties about the cancer. Others may feel that surgery will help to restore a failing relationship or to placate the distressed partner who may feel as if their partner is disfigured.

Think carefully about surgery and your goals about reconstruction. Sometimes results can be less than favorable; sometimes scars can be red and irritated, and contractures of breasts do occur. If you are concerned about nipples, surgical options, such as permanent tattooing and attachable prostheses, can help.

Magnolia Myrick:

True, surgery offers no guarantees, neither physical nor emotional, so be real clear about what your goals and intentions are. On the other hand, there are worse things than having your medical insurance pay for a great breast reconstruction. I would have not the slightest qualm about that.

14. My breasts are not even? Help!

Even without disease, our bodies are not perfectly symmetrical—breasts, feet, hands, and even our faces are often not equal in size! Uneven need not be seen as bad or abnormal. Prosthetic devices can be purchased and discreetly worn within a bra; this helps clothes to fit properly.

Because concerns need to be overcome, try practicing some self-esteem exercises. Get completely undressed, and observe yourself in the mirror. Really take a good look. Often, women have never done this after surgery. Become familiar with your new body—the new scars. Touch them and feel them. Embrace the new body. Get comfortable with the new you! The new normal is now normal! Being different than before can also be sensual and sexy!

15. I miss my sexy nipples. What can I do?

Do not underestimate the nipples. Often patients and surgeons get so caught up in the cancer and its curative surgery that they neglect to discuss nipples in the sexual response. Many women find the nipples and the surrounding tissues (**areola**) to be quite sensitive, stimulating, and erotic. Many men also find their nipples erotic! With surgical removal of the nipple, a person may feel a loss in sexuality. For cosmetic reasons, some women opt for skin grafting, which can reconstruct the nipple; thus, it may appear visually similar to its appearance before cancer surgery. Others may elect to have permanent tattooing in the nipple area. Nipple prostheses can be purchased in many specialty stores, including some department stores. If nipple stimulation was an important part of your sexual lovemaking script, acknowledge and accept this loss. Recognize that the human body has an abundant nerve supply and countless erotic and sensual areas, some of which you may yet experience.

Explore different body areas: some women enjoy having the neck, eyelids, arm creases, underarms, legs, or feet caressed and explored. Others may enjoy fingers or toes being caressed or sucked! You may be very surprised to discover that you have many undiscovered sexually charged and erotic areas on your body. Begin sexual exploration and self-discovery!

16. Why are surgeons advising me to remove my other breast?

Some women who have breast cancer may be at an increased risk for developing breast cancer in the unaffected breast. They may choose to undergo another

Areola

The circular patch of darker skin that surrounds the nipple. It is present in men and women.

You may be very surprised to discover that you have many undiscovered sexually charged and erotic areas on your body. Begin sexual exploration and self-discovery!

TREATMENTS

Thermography

Diagnostic technique using a thermograph to record the heat produced by different parts of the body; used to study blood flow and to detect tumors.

Prophylactic mastectomy

Removal of the unaffected breast tissue.

surgery rather than increased surveillance with mammograms, magnetic resonance imaging, or **thermography**. When breast cancer survivors undergo **prophylactic mastectomy** (removal of the unaffected breast tissue) and reconstruction after breast removal (sometimes with saline/water or silicone implants), sometimes the new breast may not be acceptable. Poor cosmetic results, including scarring and changes in how the breasts look and feel, may affect sexual enjoyment and self-image.

Surgical scarring may interfere with mobility, especially with arm movement. In fact, even putting an arm around their partner is painful because of lymphedema and decreased range of motion. Also, finding a comfortable sexual position may be challenging. Discuss the pros and cons about prophylactic surgery with your surgeon, your partner, your oncological team, and your sexual healthcare provider. Do not feel rushed when making a huge decision regarding a major surgical intervention.

17. What is a risk-reducing oophorectomy, and will it affect my sex life?

Bilateral salpingo-oophorectomy

The surgical term for the removal of both the right and left fallopian tubes and ovaries.

Women with breast cancer who have a genetic predisposition for the development of ovarian cancer because of *BRCA* gene mutations may opt to undergo a risk-reducing **bilateral salpingo-oophorectomy,** or voluntary removal of the ovaries. This may have negative sexual consequences. In fact, research shows that anxiety about a second malignancy in some women is not eliminated when the ovaries are removed!

Younger women who remove their ovaries may also have menopausal syndrome, including hot flashes, vaginal dryness leading to sexual pain syndromes, irritability, and mood changes. Researchers are now concerned about long-term negative health effects, such as bone health and cardiovascular disease, for these women. Have an honest discussion with your healthcare team about your risk for another breast cancer and/or ovarian cancer.

If you are at high risk for developing another cancer, you can be screened closely by your survivorship professional, your gynecology, or oncological provider. Many large hospitals have high-risk screening programs and have access to the latest technology. For ovarian cancer screening, the patient is asked to have a pelvic examination, a CA 125 blood hormone test, and a transvaginal examination. Although these tests lack considerable sensitivity and specificity, they are the best screening techniques available.

18. My scars are large, red, and ugly. What can I do?

Sometimes surgery can leave large, unsightly, or red scars; most take approximately 1 year to heal. If you scar terribly, discuss your concerns with your provider. Also, give yourself some time to heal naturally. Many surgeons and plastic surgeons advocate the use of Scarguard or Maderma, which are applied to the surgical scar site approximately 4 weeks after surgery. These medications are applied like nail polish twice daily. They may also help the **erythema** to decrease in intensity. Ask your surgeon about these products.

If after a considerable time the scars are still unsightly, tight, or uncomfortable, ask for a plastic surgery consultation, as sometimes the scar can be revised and removed. Sometimes fibrosis, or hardening and thickening of

Erythema

Redness following surgical procedure or local irritation.

the tissues, can occur. Also, physical therapy can help to stretch the area. Other women have benefited from direct injection of medications into the scar area. Help is available.

Magnolia Myrick:

This may sound funny, but I have become friends with my scar. I do look at it, touch it, and consider it. It changes subtly according to how well I'm taking care of myself. When I'm stressed or overdoing, it becomes darker and slightly irritated; when I'm in balance, it is lighter in color and pain free. I've learned to respect what the scar is "telling" me and to honor it by getting myself back on course, back in balance. My scar is a teacher and a symbol as well of my battle, my courage, and my resolve. I can't control anything "out there," but I can take each moment as it comes and be present to that. This is the deal I have with my scar.

19. My scars are erotic. Am I normal?

Yes, scars can be erotic, and the area may have heightened sensitivity. Having concern about your scar being erotic is also normal. Discuss your concerns with your provider and your partner! You have discovered a new sexual and exciting part of your body—embrace, rather than fight, the feelings. Each touch may feel different, so remember to teach your partner about what types of touch feel sexy and what types are unwelcome or painful. With education, your partner may be excited about your new-found erogenous area.

20. My husband hasn't made any effort to see me naked since the surgery? Why?

Many women and their partners are shy about exploring their bodies after surgery, chemotherapy, or radiation. There may be heightened sense of fear about the unknown. A woman should get familiar with her new body, including missing breasts and scars. Look in the mirror at the new you. Embracing the changes is often the first step toward self-acceptance! If you are uncomfortable around your partner, try sexy lingerie or some other type of revealing coverings. Take new experiences slowly. Communicate openly. If you have hit a road block, professional counseling may be needed. Often couples gradually return to sexual function, but sometimes the progress is slow and steady. There is no guideline about how long it will take you and your partner to become comfortable with your new body or scars. Every woman's experience of cancer is unique and different. Seek help if necessary.

Many women and their partners are shy about exploring their bodies after surgery, chemotherapy, or radiation.

Magnolia Myrick:

Fortunately, this wasn't an issue for me, but I realize it is for others. I asked a male friend who had divorced in his 50s and dated about seventy-two thousand women until he remarried a few years later. Yes, he said that he had been with women who had had both single and double mastectomies, some with reconstruction and some without. "Look," he said, "that has nothing to do with being sexy. Being sexy is all in the mind. It's an attitude." He could not have been more emphatic about it. "And if a mastectomy bothers him, then he's wrong." All righty then, and I agree wholeheartedly. Now if you're dating him, tell him that you need to work through the problem and seek therapy, and/or maybe you just need to move on! If you're married to him, you've got to get resolution. He might need counseling. Ask your doctor and your friends (or have him ask) if there are sexual therapists who have experience with cancer and body-image issues.

21. Which radiation-related side effects can impact my sexual desire?

Some side effects of radiation therapy include loss of hair on the scalp and/or in the genital area and diarrhea, nausea, and vomiting. Some women may lose their eye lashes and eyebrows. Obviously, if you are having specific complaints, you may not feel sexy or in the mood for sexual activity. Sometimes fatigue or exhaustion will prevail, and you'll need to rest, which is the most self-nurturing thing you can do.

Postradiation symptoms can individually or cumulatively contribute to a lack of libido or interest in physical intimacy and a sense of feeling "unsexy."

Postradiation symptoms can individually or cumulatively contribute to a lack of libido or interest in physical intimacy and a sense of feeling "unsexy." The side effects of radiation are often self-limiting and subside after treatment has been completed.

As with any cancer treatment, sexual communication between the survivor and her partner is important. A woman's partner may often feel "helpless" to assist through the difficulties of radiation therapy. He or she may welcome the opportunity to comfort her through any means (offering ice chips, assisting with the children, etc.); this can demonstrate intimacy in a variety of nonsexual ways.

22. What if I'm too fatigued from my treatment to think about sex?

Periods of intense fatigue often accompany radiation therapy. Fatigue often begins after several weeks of treatment and can last for several weeks or months after radiation has been completed. Loss of energy is temporary and need not be disabling. Cope with this by napping and going to bed earlier.

One very active woman described the period when she received radiation for breast cancer as "pure hell." She related the experience of lying in bed, completely drained of energy and vitality, while her partner silently held her in a "spoon position." This was their "sex" for the weeks of radiation treatment. His quiet support during this difficult time contributed to her feelings of connectedness to him and sexual desire for him after completion of radiation.

Give yourself some time to manage the treatments. Allow yourself time to rest, and let sexual expression take on new forms, like hugging. Sexual activity may be limited for a short time, but so are radiation treatments. Give yourself the opportunity to be tired and cope with your cancer treatments. Set limits, and learn to say no. Sometimes "toughing it out and fighting through fatigue" is not the correct answer.

Magnolia Myrick:

Yes. There were certainly times when I was tired. And while I did not push myself unreasonably, I did convince myself to keep moving—even if at a snail's pace, even if it was 20 minutes of easy-as-pie yoga, even if it was a walk around the block, even if I totally didn't feel like it. I always felt better afterward. Simple exercises for balance and flexibility are two important components of fitness, particularly as we age, and they don't require a great deal of exertion. The benefits are worth the effort. For me, yoga is a great solution. It can be active or gentle, long or short, depending on how I'm feeling that day. I also find yoga makes me feel more "in my body," and that definitely makes me feel sexier. I still can't touch the floor without bending my knees, but the last time I checked I didn't need to do that to have great sex.

Sexual activity may be limited for a short time, but so are radiation treatments. Give yourself the opportunity to be tired and cope with your cancer treatments.

23. How does radiation affect the skin on my breast? Will these changes be a turnoff to my partner?

Radiation therapy may cause redness, dryness, thickening, contractures, or changes in skin colors or texture. Expert sources at WebMD suggest that it is normal for the redness and sensitivity to persist for up to 1 year after therapy. In addition to being uncomfortable, these changes can affect a woman's body image and desire to have her breasts caressed during sexual activity.

A woman should tell her partner if her breast(s) is uncomfortably sensitive and that she is not avoiding his or her caress. Some women assume that skin changes will be a turnoff to their partners and thus avoid sexual play that involves nudity and/or touching of the breasts. Remember to explore openly, and *never* assume a partner's reaction to breast skin changes. Also, a woman may overestimate the negative impact of skin color and texture changes on her partner's sexual desire.

Conversely, if skin changes adversely affect the ongoing body image and sexual desire of either partner, the couple can address this in therapy. Your radiation oncologist can suggest medical intervention to lessen the irritation.

24. Will radiation in the nipple area decrease sensation and arousal?

Each woman reacts uniquely to radiation therapy. During therapy, some women might experience slight stinging and flakiness in the nipple. Some complain of nipple hypersensitivity, whereas others experience hyposensitivity. Communicate with a partner about any changes in nipple sensitivity. Remember that how the nipples feel immediately after radiation therapy may be different after time has passed.

If after recovery you have experienced decreased sensitivity in the nipple area, some sexual interventions can be used. Dr. Krychman and Dr. Kellogg Spadt have implemented Zestra Feminine Arousal Fluid (Semprae Laboratories), which increases sensual sensation after it is applied. Apply this fluid daily to the nipples to improve sensitivity and feeling. Excellent clinical results have been seen. Understanding what feels good and what doesn't are also important. Maintain your intimate connection to your body. Sexual exploration, even after treatment, is important. Your sexual experience may be always changing.

Magnolia Myrick:

I find the nipple on the breast where I had surgery is more sensitive, and not necessarily in a good way. The breast itself is more sensitive and a little painful at times, and I ask my partner to be very gentle there. When I asked a doctor about it—this was about a year after diagnosis and surgery— he said it might be because of nerves that were cut during surgery, etc., etc., and then he said, "It's always going to bother you." And somehow knowing that makes it bother me less because I'm not as paranoid about every little twitch. I also restrict my caffeine intake, which I have done since being diagnosed with fibrocystic breasts in my 20s. Caffeine aggravates fibrocystic breast tissue in some women, and I'm one of them. De-caffing definitely helps here.

Can't wait to try Zestra on nipples. Woo-hoo!

25. When I am receiving radiation therapy, am I radioactive? Is it dangerous to be near my partner?

Women and/or their partners may have unfounded concerns regarding being "radioactive" after radiation therapy.

Women and/or their partners may have unfounded concerns regarding being "radioactive" after radiation therapy. You cannot "catch" radiation, nor is a person "radioactive" after having undergone radiation. Maintain open communication with your partner. Sometimes the silence can be deafening. Often, cancer and its therapies can lead to miscommunication and misinterpretation.

26. What are the side effects of chemotherapy?

Menopause

The lack of menstrual cycles for one year; the permanent end of a woman's menstrual cycle.

Many agents can cause nausea, diarrhea, and mucus membrane irritation and induce premature **menopause** (no menstrual periods for 12 months) including hot flashes and vaginal dryness or atrophy. Loss of hair on the head, eyebrows, eyelashes, and hair on the genitals may be distressing and may affect a female's perception of sexual attractiveness. A smooth genital area is often looked on as prepubescent and unattractive—nonsexual.

Chemotherapy-induced early ovarian failure from surgical removal of the ovaries or from adjunctive radiation therapy can cause menopausal symptoms. Hot flashes, sleep instability, vaginal dryness, and mood problems also affect desire and arousal. Vaginal dryness can lead to painful intercourse or penetration. Many of these direct and indirect effects from chemotherapy can affect the sexual response cycle.

Healthcare providers are getting better at dosing chemotherapy. Premedications can decrease nausea and vomiting;

thus, many women who are undergoing chemotherapy do not feel ill, and many want to maintain sexual intimacy even in the face of disease. Chemotherapy-induced **vaginal dyspareunia** or chemotherapy-induced painful sex can be a result of certain medications. The chemotherapy drugs kill rapidly dividing cells, including the vaginal lining; thus, some women who are receiving active chemotherapy treatments may suffer from painful sex as a result. Minimally absorbed local vaginal estrogen products, moisturizers, and lubricants may be helpful. Discuss with your healthcare team the best healthcare treatment plan.

Vaginal dyspareunia

Pain in the vaginal area during intercourse.

TREATMENTS

27. How can I overcome my pain?

For sexuality to occur, pain control is important. Living in constant chronic pain can negatively affect the quality of life. Activities of your daily living, as well as your overall mental, physical, and emotional well-being, are impacted. Many cancer patients incorrectly believe that they need to suffer in silence. Most cancer pain can be effectively controlled. You will be able to enjoy life again, sleep better, enjoy social connections, and eat healthy after your pain is controlled. Pain that is out of control often leads to anger, frustration, **depression**, isolation, and stress.

Most cancer pain can be effectively controlled.

Pain control often involves your cancer (oncology) doctors, nurses, pharmacists, anesthesiologists, neurologists, and perhaps a specialist in pain management. Do not suffer in silence, believing that your discomfort is a sign of weakness or that your suffering is part of the healing process. Your healthcare team members can treat your pain only when they know that it exists.

Depression

A state of lowered mood usually associated with other disturbances like sleep, appetite, and loss of life's pleasure. Serious cases may be associated with suicidal thoughts.

Sometimes patients worry that they will become addicted to prescribed pain medications. This is unlikely, however, even with strong medications such as narcotics or opioids. Some people fear the potential side effects, including constipation, nausea and vomiting, lightheadedness, confusion, or a loss of control. Your doctor can modify the medications to minimize side effects while maximizing pain control.

Types of cancer pain include acute, chronic, and breakthrough pain. Pain can come from the cancer tumor or as a result of the surgery, chemotherapy, or radiation therapy. Phantom pain can occur at the site of an amputation or limb removal, and some women who have had mastectomies feel abnormal pain, sensations, or discomfort where the breast is missing.

Cancer Pain Treatments

Medications and nonmedical techniques can minimize your pain. Develop and implement an adequate pain management plan with your healthcare team.

Keep a diary to document your pain levels and quality throughout the day. Place intensity on a scale from 1 to 10, where 10 is the worst and 1 or 0 is pain free. Mark the type of pain. Is it dull? Throbbing? Sharp? Constant? What makes your pain better or worse? Also, keep record of how your pain is managed (e.g., medication and other techniques).

Some pain medications are over the counter. Before your medical visit, write a list (or bring) all of your medications. These drugs can be analyzed so that possible side effects or drug interactions can be minimized.

According to the American Cancer Society's guide on pain management, these are important questions to ask your physician before taking pain medications:

- How much medication should I take? What is the dose?
- How often should I take it?
- Can I take more if I am still in pain? How long before the medication begins working? If I can take more, how much? If no, then how long do I have to wait before the next dose?
- Should I take the medication with food or on an empty stomach?
- Can I drink alcohol with this medication? What foods should be avoided?
- Can I work, drive, or operate machinery while taking this medication?
- How does this medication interact with the other medications that I am already taking?
- What are the common side effects? How can I prevent or treat them?
- Does this medication interact with certain foods, herbs, or vitamins?
- What do I do if I run out of my prescription? What is your office practice for renewing medications?
- Is this covered by my insurance? Can I take a less expensive generic form?

The following is a list, although not exhaustive, of new mediations that may be offered. Pain medications can be pills, suppositories, patches, liquid, or injected into your bloodstream, muscle, or space around nerve endings in your spine.

- *Nonopioids.* Acetaminophen, aspirin, ibuprofen, and other nonsteroidal anti-inflammatory drugs fit into this category. Gastrointestinal upset can occur with these. Some are over the counter. Stronger doses of these types of medications may require a doctor's prescription.

- *Opioids.* This category includes morphine, fentanyl, Demerol, codeine, and oxycodone. Some of the more likely side effects of the opioids include drowsiness, constipation, nausea, or vomiting. Some people may experience itchiness over their body, confusion, or hallucinations. Opioids can be addictive. When you no longer need opioids, gradually diminish your dose and times of taking this type of medication to avoid rapid withdrawal symptoms, including generally feeling bad, a flu-like syndrome, disturbed sleep, preoccupation with physical symptoms, and a lower threshold for tolerating stress. These symptoms may go away in a short time in healthy individuals.

- *Antidepressants and anticonvulsants.* These can be used for pain that causes burning or tingling. **Antidepressants** can treat mood disorders as well as chronic pain syndromes. Common side effects include dry mouth, a drop in blood pressure, an inability to urinate, or drowsiness.

Antidepressant

The best medication to treat depression and panic attacks. They are nonaddictive and may benefit the central nervous system in many ways.

"Holding off" between doses is counterproductive in controlling your pain. Taking your medications at a fixed time may be the best method to control your cancer pain effectively. If you experience any side effects or complications from your medications, seek professional medical advice. Your physician can help you manage these side effects or can change your medication entirely.

A number of strategies, including hypnosis, biofeedback, guided imagery, acupuncture, deep rhythmic breathing, or physical therapy, can help you to cope with pain and anxiety. Many comprehensive cancer institutions have a department of alternative or complementary medicine or know about resources where these services can be provided. If you suffer from chronic pain, seek some emotional counseling or supportive care. Other specialized techniques such as **reflexology, Shiatsu massage, aromatherapy, Reiki, meditation**, and **yoga** may also be helpful for pain control.

Minimize your pain level before considering sexual activity.

28. What is menopause, and what can I expect? My vagina and vulva hurt and burn. What can I do?

In menopause, a woman does not have a menstrual cycle for 1 year. A woman may go through natural menopause, where her cycles stop spontaneously, usually around age of 51 years. Natural menopause is as a result of a variety of factors such as genetics, smoking, and age of first menstrual cycle. Chemical menopause occurs when the woman has received chemicals (like chemotherapy) or medications that temporarily or permanently stop her menstrual cycles. Some prescription medications, such as a gonadotropin releasing hormone agonist, shut down her pituitary gland and ovaries, decreasing the signaling hormones, like follicle stimulating hormone and luteinizing hormone, that stimulate the ovaries. This may thereby create a menopausal state. Surgical menopause is when both ovaries are removed; thus, hormones are no longer produced.

In the menopausal transition, the vulva and the vagina can change in overall appearance and texture. The menopausal period is often accompanied by vaginal dryness and other changes in the **perineal area**. The vulva, vagina, and clitoris can become very dry, irritated, and even sore as a result of falling estrogen levels. The vagina

Reflexology

A therapeutic method of relieving pain by stimulating predefined pressure points on the feet and hands.

Shiatsu massage

A manipulative therapy developed in Japan and incorporating techniques of anma (Japanese traditional massage), acupressure, stretching, and Western massage. Shiatsu involves applying pressure to special points or areas on the body in order to maintain physical and mental well being, treat disease, or alleviate discomfort.

Aromatherapy

An integrative care practice that uses oils from plants to treat physical or psychological conditions. The oils can be inhaled, used in vaporizers, or used in massage.

Reiki

A form of therapy that uses simple hands-on, no-touch, and visualization techniques, with the goal of improving the flow of life energy in a person.

TREATMENTS

Meditation

A complementary medicine practice of concentrated attention toward a single point of reference.

Yoga

The spiritual practice aiming to unite the consciousness with universal consciousness to achieve harmony.

Perineal area

The genital area between the vulva and anus.

may become frail, pale, and less elastic; urinary tract infections may become more common. Other women may also complain of increased time to achieve orgasm or decreased orgasmic intensity. To prevent or minimize pain, itching, redness, or burning, skin care of the vulva is important. Changes can be minimized, and minor alterations in perineal and vulvar hygiene can help prevent further damage to the sensitive area of the pelvis. Breathable clothing (e.g., cotton) should minimize vaginal or vulvar irritation. At home, some women may prefer not to wear underwear at all. Wear thigh- or knee-high hose instead of pantyhose. If you must wear pantyhose, try cutting out the center of the crotch because tight-fitting underwear can cause increased discomfort. Choose loose-fitting pants or skirts, and remember to remove wet bathing suits and exercise clothing promptly.

Some suggestions to help maintain healthy vulvar and vaginal health are listed here:

- Use only mild detergents to wash undergarments and underwear. Double rinse underwear and any other clothing that comes into contact with the vulva. Do not use a fabric softener. Minimize the amount of chemicals that are left over in any clothing.

- Use soft, white, unscented toilet paper. Pat the vulvar area dry with light pressure only. Do not rub; this can create a scratching irritation.

- Some women use lukewarm or cool baths to relieve irritation. Fill your bath with only 1 or 2 inches of tepid water. Adding four to five tablespoons of baking soda, colloidal oatmeal (such as Aveeno), or even chamomile tea bags to the water may help reduce itching and irritation.

- Abstain from a perfumed bubble bath, creams, sprays or soaps, and feminine hygiene products. Avoid lotions in the pelvic area. Do not spray perfume in the genital area.

- Use a soft cloth or your fingers to cleanse the vulva. Wash the vulva with cool to lukewarm water only. If you feel you must use soap, use soap for sensitive skin that is mild and unscented. Pat the area dry gently with a soft towel. Some use a *cool* hair dryer at a distance from the genital area to help keep the area dry.

- Rinse the vulva area completely after urination (possibly with a small spray bottle filled with cool tap water). Urinate often before your bladder is completely full.

- If you are menstruating, be sure to use 100% cotton menstrual pads and tampons. Caracara and Organic Essentials may be helpful, but others may also be on the market.

Be careful when shaving or trimming pubic hair. Sometimes ingrown hairs or the act of shaving, waxing, or cutting hair can increase the irritation in the genitals. Be especially careful at menopause when the vaginal and vulvar regions are extra sensitive.

This list contains a few tips that you can follow to help you maintain vaginal health:

- Avoid strenuous exercises such as bicycle riding and horseback riding that can put direct pressure on the vulvar tissues. Be careful to change your clothes after the activity, and try to limit the time you are engaged in these activities.

- Limit any intense exercise that creates a lot of friction in the vulvar area, especially those that cause

Labia majora

Outer vaginal lips.

Labia minora

Inner vaginal lips.

the **labia majora** and **labia minora** to rub against one another. Attempt to slow the intensity of exercises such as walking.

- Use a frozen gel pack (or maybe even frozen peas in a plastic bag wrapped in a towel) wrapped in a towel to relieve symptoms after exercise. Wash and dry the genitals completely after vigorous exercise and perspiration.

- Enroll in yoga to learn stretching and relaxation exercises.

- Limit the time you spend swimming in highly chlorinated pools, and avoid soaking in hot tubs or very hot baths. After swimming, be sure to shower after a swim or soak to limit exposure to harsh chemicals.

- By drinking plenty of fluids, you will help keep your urine diluted and less likely to sting or irritate the vulvar area.

- Ask your healthcare provider whether you should use a foam rubber donut if you are sitting for long periods.

- If you must sit all day, try to alternate periods of standing and exercise throughout the day.

Vaginal atrophy

When the vaginal tissues decrease in size and become pale or dry without lubrication, this is a result of decreased hormonal levels in the woman's body. The tissues can become sensitive, and often vaginal atrophy is associated with painful intercourse. This is commonly seen in chemical or natural menopause.

Dry Vagina

Vaginal tissues naturally become dry as a woman's estrogen levels decrease. This can lead to itchiness, burning, irritation, and often painful intercourse. Luckily, many methods can treat the symptoms of vaginal dryness or **vaginal atrophy**. As women age, the vagina becomes dry and less elastic. Cancer treatments can hasten these changes. Some women can take estrogen either by a pill, patch, cream, ring, or gel to prevent these changes; however, these may not be safe options for many women who have had breast cancer, especially those with hormonally sensitive cancers. Review the suggestions listed in this section with your healthcare provider before considering estrogen therapy.

Many products on the market may help maintain your vaginal moisture. A simple vitamin E capsule can be punctured with a pin and then inserted into your vagina. (If you insert the entire capsule into the vagina, the gel cap will come out in time.) You can also empty the capsule's content onto your finger and insert vaginally. Replens, Me Again, and Feminease can be purchased over the counter and come with easily filled applicators. You can use any of these moisturizers two to three times a week. These and other moisturizers are readily available without a prescription in most drug stores or via the Internet. Remember that you may need to wear a panty liner. If you also use a vaginal estrogen product, alternate the days you use a moisturizer. For example, use the moisturizer on Monday, Wednesday, and Friday and the local estrogen product on Tuesday, Thursday, and Saturday. Some of the moisturizers contain bactericides, spermicidal components, colors, flavors, and other additives that irritate the sensitive vaginal lining. Avoid additives such as parabens and glycerin, which promote infections and in some cases act as drying agents. Vaginal moisturizers should be used on a regular basis, independently of sexual intercourse, as they hydrate the vaginal lining and restore vaginal elasticity.

Vaginal lubricants (Slippery Stuff, Hydra, YES Eros Woman, Astroglide, and KY Jelly) are typically used to make sexual intercourse more pleasurable. Organically made choices are Good Clean Love and Almost Naked. These are made with natural ingredients and are quite comfortable and effective. These are organic, free of parabens and glycerin products, and extra gentle for the delicate vaginal and vulvar tissues. For more information on their products contact *www.goodcleanlove.com*.

A good lubricant is water based and compatible with diaphragms or condoms. Once applied, they stay moist without becoming sticky, goopy, or gummy. They are typically easy to apply and easy to clean. Because each has a different consistency, experiment with different types to determine which feels best during intercourse. Many can be purchased at your local grocery store or over the Internet. Menopausal women with severe vaginal atrophy and thinning of the vaginal lining should avoid irritating additives such as colors, flavors, spermicidal additives, bactericides, or warming ingredients. Mineral oil, petroleum jelly, and edible oils or other liquid food products can sometimes be effectively used on the vulva but should be generally avoided within the vaginal canal. Oils can upset the delicate balance between the good and bad bacteria and thus possibly result in vaginal infections. Also, these products have also been known to reduce the safety of condoms.

Local vaginal hormones come in a variety of different application methods. Creams, gels, rings, and tablets are the most common. Vaginal and vulvar creams like Premarin Vaginal Cream (Pfizer Pharmaceuticals) or Estrace Cream (Warner Chicott) are typically applied to both the interior of the vagina and exterior of the vulvar vault. Premarin Vaginal Cream recently became the first and only medication that is Food and Drug Administration (FDA) approved for the treatment of moderate to severe painful intercourse. Premarin Cream contains conjugated equine estrogens and is readily available; new lowered doses demonstrate excellent safety on the endometrial lining. Estrace Cream contains **estradiol**, which is also helpful for treatment of vulvovaginal atrophy and sexual pain. Many women find these especially soothing, and those with extreme vulvar atrophy and shrinkage may benefit from these. Creams are helpful when considering

Estradiol

The predominant sex hormone present in females.

treatment for vulvar dryness and clitoral shrinkage and atrophic changes. Both Dr. Kellogg Spadt and Dr. Krychman have used this medication when women with breast cancer complain of orgasmic changes, as ultra small amounts of cream can be rubbed into the clitoral area with substantial orgasmic changes. Of course, estrogen use in women with breast cancer or a history of a hormonally sensitive tumor is controversial and should be discussed with their healthcare team.

The ring, Estring (Pfizer Pharmaceuticals), which is used within the vaginal vault for 3 months and then is replaced, does not work as a medical device used for pelvic floor defects and does not help with urinary incontinence. Some women use the ring because they do not have to remember to use a product on a daily basis and it is minimally absorbed; however, others find it uncomfortable, and some partners feel the ring during intercourse.

Minimally absorbed vaginal tablets, Vagifem (Novo-Nordisk Pharmaceuticals), are another type of vaginal hormone replacement. Vagifem tablets are contained in a plastic disposable applicator. Insert a tablet it into your vagina every night for 14 days; then insert it twice a week at bedtime. This medication contains 17β-estradiol and comes in convenient prefilled, biodegradable applicators. A small and controversial study in the United Kingdom reported increased estradiol levels in the women using Vagifem. Many women prefer Vagifem because there is no mess or leakage, and it is easy to use. The long-term safety for minimally absorbed vaginal estrogen products needs to be further studied, especially in larger populations. A new effective ultralow dose of Vagifem is also available.

The safety of minimally absorbed local estrogen products in the breast cancer population appears (but has not been

39

Progesterone

A hormone that is secreted by the ovary and placenta (during pregnancy). It is necessary for pregnancy and has been implicated in female sexual function.

proven) to be good. The need for a **progesterone** agent if you are only on a minimally absorbed vaginal product is controversial. Some healthcare providers advocate a progesterone agent in women with an intact uterus. Of course, any abnormal vaginal bleeding should always be reported, and an immediate comprehensive workup (may include a transvaginal ultrasound and or endometrial biopsy) should be performed. Ask your doctor, nurse practitioner, or other sexual medicine specialists, and make an individualized personalized treatment plan for your vaginal and vulvar dryness.

29. My appearance has changed. I don't even look or feel like myself. What is the Look Good…Feel Better Program? How can I deal with my new body image?

The Look Good…Feel Better Program is a free service provided so that women with cancer can learn new ways to restore body image and cope with the changes in appearance. This exciting program is a joint venture between the American Cancer Society, the Cosmetic, Toiletry and Fragrance Association Foundation, and the National Cosmetology Association. Certified skin, nail care, and hair specialists, as well as professional makeup artists, educate the cancer survivor about new techniques to enhance her physical image. The information provided on the next page was taken from the American Cancer Society website.

Sometimes physical appearance can be linked with self-esteem. Women who have breast cancer surgery may have a different shape and/or altered appearance to their breasts. With complete mastectomies and

Look Good ... Feel Better

Group workshops are available: Volunteer beauty professionals lead small groups, usually about 6 to 10 women, through practical, hands-on experience. Women learn about makeup, skin care, nail care, and ways to deal with hair loss such as with wigs, turbans, and scarves. Each woman gets a free makeup kit to use during and after the workshop.

One-on-one salon consultations: Services are available for patients who are unable to go to a group workshop. A free, one-time, individual salon consultation with a volunteer cosmetologist may be available in their area. These trained beauty experts help each patient manage her skin, nail, and hair needs and also help her find ways to feel better about how she looks during treatment. Free self-help materials can be ordered through the Look Good ... Feel Better toll-free number, 1-800-395-LOOK (1-800-395-5665). The self-help materials include a 30-minute video entitled *Just for You: A Step-by-Step Guide to Help You Look Good and Feel Better During Cancer Treatment*, a step-by-step instructional booklet and an evaluation form. The videotape features cancer survivors and volunteers talking about the ways cancer treatment and side effects can affect the way you look. It also covers detailed skin care information, "how to" makeup tips, wig information, and pointers on head coverings. The booklet that goes with the video also covers nail care. Materials are also offered in Spanish, and bilingual programs are available in some areas.

chest wall radiation, the resulting chest may appear disfigured. Surgical reconstruction may not change how a woman feels about her breasts and changed appearance. The survivor may feel ashamed, embarrassed, or worried about getting undressed in front of her partner, as emotional rejection is a concern. A woman can regain a sense of femininity while maintaining high fashion. In association with self-esteem exercises and perhaps

Chest wall radiation

Radiation to the chest.

41

psychological counseling, she can choose from an array of bras, lingerie, and sportswear.

Fashionable, stylish clothes can help a woman to reclaim a sense of beauty and help her to feel attractive.

Fashionable, stylish clothes can help a woman to reclaim a sense of beauty and help her to feel attractive. A woman may experience grief when she feels that she is no longer the same person physically. She may also grieve that she is no longer able to have more children. The appendix lists many resources to women to cope with body image and to regain self-esteem. Also, sexy lingerie is available for those who have had mastectomies or lumpectomies. Nottiwear, a Canadian company, specializes in this type of sensual lingerie; see *www.nottiwear.com*.

Ostomy

A bag that is on the outside of the body used to store fecal waste in the event of a urine, colonic, or anal resection.

Some women who have an **ostomy** (a bag that is on the outside of the body used to store fecal waste in the event of a colonic or anal resection) may be self-conscious about the appearance and are concerned about foul odors and spillage. This may limit her ability to pursue new friendships and sexual relationships. These suggestions might help women with an ostomy bag: purchasing lingerie specifically designed as ostomy covers and changing the ostomy bag frequently, in anticipation of social situations or sexual activity. In addition, specially designed, odor-controlling tablets can be placed in the bag to minimize offensive odors. Certain foods that may cause increased odors should be avoided as well. During sexual activity, remember to liberally use pillows and comforters. Choose sexual positions that are comfortable and that place minimal pressure on your ostomy bag.

Magnolia Myrick:

Go ahead, girl, be a "cancer vixen." Treat yourself to that lingerie and love it. You probably needn't limit yourself to "special" lingerie shops; however, you may find wider selections at regular lingerie shops and do a bit of creative adaptation if necessary. Cancer Vixen, *by the way, is an uproarious memoir by Marisa Acocella Marchetto about her breast cancer diagnosis and treatment. She pulls no punches and it's a great read.*

30. What can I do since I have lost all my hair?

Some women spend many hours brushing, blow drying, styling, and coloring their hair, so it can be devastating when hair loss is a part of your cancer survivorship. According to the American Academy of Dermatology, by the age of 40, approximately 40% of women have begun to experience some form of hair loss. Hair problems include **hirsutism** (excessive hair growth on the face) and **alopecia** (loss of hair on the scalp). For some women, hair loss can be all-over thinning. Because of menopause and lowered estrogen levels, chronic thinning of your existing hair pattern can be seen, especially on the top of the scalp or frontal area.

Hirsutism
Excessive hair growth.

Alopecia
Loss of hair.

Some women may benefit from women's minoxidil (Rogaine) (McNeil Pharmaceuticals), a topical medication that may stimulate hair follicle growth and increase blood circulation to the scalp. Common side effects include itchiness of the scalp, headache, heart palpitations, and mild facial hair growth. Another oral medical hair-loss treatment, Finasteride (Propecia) (Merck), is presently not indicated and approved for the treatment of women with alopecia. An herbal product, Revivogen, may promote hair growth and prevent further loss or thinning. Hair transplantation is a surgical procedure that moves hair follicles from one area to another. Wigs are another practical suggestion for women who have had hair loss. They are no longer the plastic, fake-looking

TREATMENTS

43

hairpieces of the past, but are very well made and are able to be colored, styled, and personalized. Well-constructed wigs can be discreet, stylish, and natural looking. You can do most activities without fear that they will fall off. Wigs are low maintenance and flexible.

Several nonprofit organizations, such as Locks of Love, collect human hair donations so that wigs can be manufactured for cancer survivors. This group provides hairpieces to financially disadvantaged children across the United States. These children receive custom-made wigs for free or on a sliding-scale based on need. Wigs for Kids, another nonprofit group, also gives hairpieces to children.

For more information concerning the services that are available in your area or if you would like to enhance your physical appearance, contact the Look Good…Feel Better Organization (*www.lookgoodfeelbetter.org*).

Magnolia Myrick:

Hair loss can be devastating, but it does grow back. And meanwhile I do not have to spend hours (and hours) fooling with it to make it look good or paying somebody to make it look good. I see (and saw) this as a bonus. It almost made up for the time spent going to doctors' appointments and treatments and radiation and all that—not quite, but almost.

Wigs are great. They really are. The fake-hair ones now are really good. Everyone told me if I got an expensive, custom-made, real-hair wig and a less expensive good fake that I would end up wearing the fake one most of the time. I didn't believe it, but they were right. Wish I had saved myself the thousands the fancy one cost and just gone with the several hundred-dollar fake. There are also in-betweens—wigs that are combinations of real and artificial hair, with varying prices in the hundreds, generally. Check the Internet and

Yellow Pages. Go to the wig place and try them on. Have them cut, color, and style it especially for you. That's what they do.

Near the end of treatment, I got a shorter wig to make the transition to my real hair less dramatic.

When you do begin sporting your real hair again, have it professionally cut and shaped. Mine was dark and curly ("chemo curls" they call them) for about a year. I looked like a Kewpie Doll—or a poodle. Anyway it was cute.

I definitely kept my wig or scarf or whatever on during The Act, lest I burst into a "Kojak" impersonation at just the wrong moment. You have to be careful about swinging from the chandelier and stuff like that, but otherwise, those wigs stay on pretty well by themselves. If you use wig-tape, they aren't going anywhere, trust me. Think all those Broadway dancers are wearing their natural hair? So you can have sex and be in a kick-line while wearing a wig. I didn't usually sleep in a wig, though. Once I slept in a cute little white knit cap, and my boyfriend said it was like sleeping with the pope. We still laugh about that, but I did not tell the pope.

31. How can I manage my terrible hot flashes?

Even though many women are candidates for estrogen or a combination of estrogen and progesterone therapies, these treatments may not be an option for those who have had breast cancer. Some breast cancer survivors may decline systemic hormonal use because these hormones may trigger the regrowth of a tumor or stimulate a pre-existing cancer in the breast. These other ways can help to minimize some of the adverse effects of hot flashes:

1. Wear absorbent cotton clothing. Dress so that the outermost layers can be removed when you get a hot flash. Cotton is quick drying; its wicking effect traps and removes moisture from your body. Special sleepwear has been developed for those with night-time hot flashes (Wicking Menopause pajamas).

2. As soon as you feel a hot flash, drink an ice-cold glass of water or put a cold compress on your face. Misting bottles can help you spritz water. Running cold water on your wrists or immersing your feet in cold water can also provide relief.

3. Turn down the heat in the winter and raise the air-conditioning in the summer. It is easy for your partner to put on a sweater or sleep with a heavier blanket.

4. Use a room fan, or wave a hand-held fan. Fancy paper or fabric fans make beautiful accessories to any stylish outfit. Keep one in your purse and another in your car or office for easy access.

5. Techniques such as yoga, meditation, and Tai Chi may be helpful for troublesome hot flashes and are also helpful in decreasing stress and anxiety.

6. Research has shown that women who exercise regularly may have less difficulty with menopausal hot flashes. Start an exercise program today.

7. Avoid cigarette smoking.

8. Sleep near an open window or an air conditioning unit.

9. Change sleeping attire and bed linen to lighter fabrics. Menopausal pajamas can be special ordered online. Maybe even sleep nude!

10. Purchase a personal cooling pillow (*www.chillow .com*). It works by keeping your head cool.

11. Keep a hot-flash diary. Record the number and intensity of hot flashes each day. Show your diary to your clinician.

12. Avoid hot baths or showers in the 2 hours prior to going to bed.

13. Practice the paced respiration techniques described later here.

The way that you breathe has been shown to reduce the frequency and intensity of menopausal hot flashes. When the paced respiration technique is used correctly, hot flashes can be eased by at least 50%.

Perform these two steps to do the paced respiration:

1. Make a conscious effort to remain calm. In a relaxed manner, take six to eight slow, deep breaths through your nose. Each breath in and out should take at least 1 minute.

2. During each inhalation, allow the air to slowly enter your body, filling your abdomen first, and then your lungs, filling your body with more and more air. If you place your hand on your belly, you can feel your abdomen expand and sense your chest cavity as it widens. Exhale through your nose or mouth just as slowly and evenly, feeling your chest and abdomen as they contract.

Practice these paced respirations for at least 15 minutes for at least two times every day. In addition, this breathing exercise can be done any time day or night. It is very useful to do these breaths while waiting in the grocery store line, driving in traffic, or when you are in any type of stressful situation. Paced respirations may also be helpful

The way that you breathe has been shown to reduce the frequency and intensity of menopausal hot flashes.

in situations where in the past you have had a hot flash (e.g., being in a room that feels too warm). Paced respirations may also act to calm your mind and lessen distress and anxiety (adapted from Memorial Sloan-Kettering Cancer Center's patient educational materials).

Magnolia Myrick:

Layers, definitely, and if it is cold outside stick your head out the window or go stand outside for a minute. Open up the freezer for a quick cool jolt of fresh air!

I've also acquired a lovely little collection of fans and have found them very handy. Portable and practical, they are also quite a lot of fun and almost always conversation pieces. Not to mention fashion accessories.

32. What other techniques can I implement to help with my hot flashes?

A healthy diet is important for overall general health, fitness, and strength. Many women find some relief from menopausal hot flashes with some minor dietary changes and/or the addition of some basic vitamin and mineral supplements. Moderation is the key when making any changes to your food intake. Avoid certain triggers that may include caffeine, alcohol (including beer, wine, and liquor), and spicy foods. Consider adding some vitamin supplements such as vitamin B6 (200 or 250 mg daily) or Peridin C (two tablets three times a day). Begin with these over-the-counter medicines, and allow at least 4 to 6 weeks for them to work. If possible, add one supplement at a time so that you can determine whether it is working for you. Complementary medicine and alternative techniques or therapies use the disciplines of modern science and medicine and couple them with ancient philosophies from different cultures.

As a result, many techniques incorporate modern Western and traditional Eastern philosophies. Many strategies have gained popularity as they can help to ease suffering and promote healing or feelings of well-being.

Many cancer survivors will use a variety of herbal supplements or other unconventional techniques to help maintain an improved quality of life or minimize troublesome side effects. Some of the more common herbal or homeopathic preparations for menopausal women include isoflavones, black cohosh, chaste tree berry, ginseng, dong quai, evening primrose oil, wild yam, motherwort, red clover, linden flower, yarrow, green tea extract, and klimaktheel. The American College of Obstetricians and Gynecologists Task Force on Hormone Therapy has examined the scientific evidence for soy, black cohosh, red clover, and Mexican progesterone yam cream for the treatment of menopausal hot flashes. Unfortunately, these products did not reduce hot flashes by a clinically significant amount, and medical literature does not conclusively support their use. Still, many perimenopausal and menopausal women have claimed that these products are effective in managing their individual menopause symptoms. There is limited scientific evidence that many herbs that are listed here significantly diminish menopausal symptoms. Results vary. The term "herbal" does not necessarily connote effective or risk free. In fact, some herbs may have potentially harmful side effects and may interact with chemotherapy and other prescribed medications. Always be cautious, and if you are considering using herbal therapy, check with your cancer specialist or clinician. Several websites discuss herbs, their medical indications, and possible interactions and effects (see Memorial Sloan-Kettering Cancer Center, *www.mskcc.org/aboutherbs*; National Center for Complementary and Alternative Medicine, *www.nccam.nih.gov*).

Alternative medicine and relaxation techniques (e.g., foot reflexology, magnet therapy, meditation, yoga, and therapeutic massage) can minimize hot flashes, although success rates are variable. Their ability to decrease the severity or even prevent hot flashes lacks scientific randomized controlled studies that prove effective.

Many women report that acupuncture relieves hot flashes.

Acupuncture

A traditional Chinese practice of treating a health condition or medical state by inserting needles into the skin at specific points to unblock the flow of energy.

Many women report that acupuncture relieves hot flashes. **Acupuncture** is the ancient Chinese medical system in which very thin needles are painlessly and strategically placed into the skin. It is used to control chronic pain and heal a variety of other ailments. Acupuncture works by stimulating specific portions of the nervous system, relieving pain by causing signal transmitters and hormones in the brain to work in different ways. Many local and national cancer institutions have excellent integrative medicine departments that specialize in herbal supplements as well as complementary and alternative medicine choices. Dr. Krychman, in association with the Healing Sanctuary, located in Southern California, has developed a menopausal and hot flash program with director and acupuncturist Pam Jacobson. Together they implement both Western and Eastern techniques with the shared goal of hot flash management. The program has been well received in Orange County among cancer patients and their treating healthcare providers. For more information, visit the Healing Sanctuary at *www.thehealingsanctuaryoc.com.*

Both Memorial Sloan-Kettering Cancer Center and the M.D. Anderson Cancer Center have excellent resources available. For more information concerning the medical uses of acupuncture, consult the American Academy of Medical Acupuncture at *www.medicalacupuncture.org.*

33. What prescription medications are helpful for hot flash management?

Many prescription medications are available to help with hot flashes. Talk with your healthcare provider to see whether you should try another type of medicine and to discuss possible side effects. Some prescription medications that can be helpful with troublesome hot flashes include the following:

- Antihypertensive mediations (e.g., clonidine and methyldopa)

- Antidepressants or the **selective serotonin reuptake inhibitors** (SSRIs) (e.g., venlafaxine [Effexor], Pfizer Pharmaceuticals; paroxetine [Paxil], GlaxoSmith-Kline Pharmaceuticals)

Studies on the SSRI medication Paxil have shown success for the treatment of moderate hot flashes. Many women find this medication very helpful in small doses, but others who may be very sensitive to this class of drugs may experience negative sexual side effects from SSRI medications. Some emerging evidence shows that this class of medication may not be advisable with women who are taking **Tamoxifen**. Consult your survivorship medicine expert or your oncologist to discuss your situation.

- Antiepileptics (e.g., gabapententin [Neurontin])

Regardless of which medication you may be trying, remember that all medications may cause side effects. In addition to discussing the drug with your clinician, carefully read the package insert, and ask about potential drug–drug interactions that may occur (including alcohol).

TREATMENTS

Selective serotonin reuptake inhibitor

A type of depressant medication that does not allow serotonin to be taken up again by the neuroreceptors, thereby causing more serotonin to be present in the neuron. These may be used for depression and panic attacks. Some include Prozac, Zoloft, Paxil, Celexa, Luvox, and Lexapro.

Tamoxifen

A selective estrogen receptor modulator that is used in the treatment of breast cancer.

34. I can't even remember what sex used to be like. Cancer has affected my mind and memory. Please help.

With certain chemotherapies, sometimes women complain of increased forgetfulness or loss of memory. You can do many things to improve your memory. Mental techniques and nutrition may help improve your short- and long-term memory.

Stimulate Your Memory

Your mind is like any other muscle in your body. You must exercise and use it for it to be strong and healthy. For example, you can learn new skills. Teach yourself a new computer software program. Take a ballroom dancing class, and practice the steps. Go to a home-improvement workshop and learn how to tile, fix plumbing, or build a deck. Begin a home project. Art classes are fun places to learn how to work clay to throw a pot, paint china, sew, or draw. Play games like chess or backgammon; do crossword puzzles or wonder words. Vary the activities that you are doing. Hobby and toy departments of your local stores sell all kinds of card and number games (such as the popular Sudoku) that allow you to exercise your number skills. Picture puzzles are a relaxing way to explore shapes and colors; crossword puzzles help you to recall words and names. Read new books on a variety of new and exciting topics. Share a movie or a newspaper article with your partner, and then discuss it. Watch a movie documentary or action adventure movie, and try to recall the details of the plot to a friend. Use your memory and help stimulate your brain cells to maintain their health!

Focus on Things Around You, and Start to Notice Every Detail!

Try to focus your attention and concentration on the issues that are most important. Address the details and concentrate. Try to maintain your focus. Consciously block out all other distractions. One interesting game is Concentration. Place common household objects like a pen, pencil, and safety pin on a tray. Notice their characteristics and texture, their distinct and defining attributes. Try to block out all other distractions as you focus on the objects. Then turn away and recall each one. When meeting new people, notice things about them, and then try to associate some detail with their name or personality. For instance, if you meet someone new named Jennifer who wears glasses and is a nuclear physicist, begin to associate her wearing glasses with her highly technical and intricate profession.

Relax and Visualize

Attention requires relaxation, so be relaxed, well rested, and in control of stress and emotions. Deep, slow, quiet breathing often can help. Take a deep breath in, and hold it for 5 to 10 seconds before slowly releasing. Breathe deeply into and out of your diaphragm. Try to see objects in your mind. Use your senses to describe the objects (taste, texture, and touch). Do this with your favorite food. Imagine your favorite restaurant or the smell of your partner's cologne or perfume.

Mnemonics and Other Memory Games

Mnemonics is an easy way to remember sequences. A special word can be used to remember something, particularly lists. Another technique is alliteration, where the same consonants are repeated in a group of words. Associate a person with an object that rhymes with his or her name. (For example, Michael has black wavy hair that seems to flow in the air when he runs, as if he were riding a motorcycle. Calling him "Motorcycle Michael" in your head may help you to remember his name.) Rhyming can help, too. These are very efficient ways to memorize large quantities of information.

Foods, Water, and Alcohol

A well-balanced diet is paramount for an excellently functioning memory. Some believe that certain vitamins, such as thiamin, folic acid, and vitamin B12, may be helpful with memory. Foods such as bread, cereal, some fruits, and vegetables contain these vitamins. Some memory experts believe that vitamins may improve memory, but other healthcare providers have their doubts. No medically sound studies have been performed that document that vitamin supplementation improves either short- or long-term memory.

According to one memory expert, Dr. Carol Truking-ton, the lack of water in the body has an immediate and deep effect on memory. Dehydration generates confusion and thought difficulties. Alcohol also interferes with short-term memory, thus impairing the ability to process and retain new information. Even drinking small quantities of an alcoholic beverage during one entire week impairs memory. Although caffeine in coffee, tea, and chocolate may help you to be attentive, excess caffeine results in a state of excitement that interferes with memory function.

Sleep

The brain and the entire human body require time to relax and recover from the stressful day's events. Adequate peaceful and deep sleep is essential for good memory skills. During sleep, the mind relaxes, revives, and rejuvenates. If you are excessively stressed or suffer from chronic exhaustion as a result of being underrested, you may also complain of having a poor memory. Chronic fatigue, emotional or physical stress, and the lack of complete rest can impair concentration and the ability of the brain to process and retain new information.

Medication

Many medications, including tranquilizers, muscular relaxants, sleeping pills, and antianxiety drugs, can contribute to the loss of memory. Also, benzodiazepines, such as diazepam (Valium) and lorazepam (Ativan), can contribute to memory problems. Antihypertensive medications that are used to control high blood pressure may not only cause sexual difficulties, but also memory changes and a depressed mood. Before discontinuing or changing dosage of medication, consult with your healthcare provider. Some medications, when stopped suddenly, can cause harmful side effects and symptoms.

Smoking

Smoking is a serious health concern, as it contributes to cancer, particularly in the lungs, mouth, and tongue. It also decreases the amount of oxygen delivered to the brain, affecting memory and cognitive functioning.

Practical Techniques to Increase My Memory

Creative memory aids, such as the following, can be used to remember important names, places, stories, and words used in your daily living.

1. *Write.* Writing takes an idea out of your mind and makes it a record that can be easily remembered. Write and review lists. Keep a personal journal of important things or events you want to remember.

If you are excessively stressed or suffer from chronic exhaustion as a result of being under-rested, you may also complain of having a poor memory.

TREATMENTS

2. *Organize.* Sort your papers, and throw away what you no longer need. Have baskets, labeled file folders, or an organizing system to sort bills, instruction manuals, and papers. Decluttering your home and office helps to calm your mind. Most people feel quite satisfied after their space has been cleaned and organized.

3. *Schedule.* Keep a calendar, and write your appointments and regular activities. Then you can review what you will do each day. When new things come up, it is easier to cluster activities or make decisions about whether you are able to do them now or later or not at all.

4. *Use notepads.* Place many notepads (each with a pen or pencil) around your home and/or office. When you want to remember something, grab your notepad and jot it down. Later, this information can be added to your calendar or filed appropriately.

5. *Use memory strategies.* Use memory-aiding techniques.

6. *Keep a shopping list.* Before you go shopping, list the items you want to purchase.

If still have concerns about your recent memory loss, then consult a memory specialist for some specific tests. Disorders in memory can disrupt your quality of life. If your memory loss is severe, it may caused by a more serious underlying medical issue, including menopause, hormonal or vitamin deficiencies, mental depression, infections, and dementias. Many memory and aging facilities specialize in assessment, diagnosis, and treatment of memory disorders. Ask your primary care physician if a referral is right for you.

35. I am too tired for sex. How can I decrease fatigue?

Fatigue is a common problem for patients with cancer and is devastating because it directly impacts your daily activities and the lives of others with whom you associate. When you are fatigued, feeling interested in sex is not on your agenda.

Common causes of fatigue include side effects of medications, underactive thyroid gland, destruction of cancer cells, infection, uncontrolled pain, fever, poor nutrition, anemia, mental depression, poor sleeping patterns, anxiety, and emotional stress. Some causes of fatigue are easily treated. Before your visit to the clinic, describe and record the times of the day when you feel most tired. Certain medications like erythropoietin (Procrit, Epogen) (Amgen) or darbepoetin (Aranesep) (Amgen) can be given by injection to women who have anemia, and these medications have been shown to help with fatigue.

According to a Memorial Sloan-Kettering handout, other helpful techniques to decrease fatigue include

- Sleep extra hours, go to bed earlier, or stay in bed later in the morning. If you are unable to sleep, you may benefit from a short course of sleep medications. Ask your healthcare provider if these are appropriate for you. Most prescriptions are short term because they can be habit forming.
- Eliminate difficult activities that cause fatigue, and pace yourself throughout the day.
- Schedule rest throughout the day.
- Ask for help from family and friends. Household chores like cooking, cleaning, and grocery shopping and child care can be delegated to family or friends.

- Do not be afraid to limit your activities and obligations. Learn to say "no," but do not isolate yourself from your social network.

- Ask your healthcare team if some of your medications could be contributing to your fatigue. If so, then discuss a substitute medication or whether you can limit your intake.

- Plan a well-balanced diet. Eat plenty of fruits and vegetables, and drink 8 to 10 glasses of water per day. Avoid caffeinated beverages or alcohol, especially in the evening hours. See a nutritionist, or consider incorporating some vitamin supplements.

- Maintain a light, tailored exercise plan. Exercise actually boosts your energy level as long as you do not overdo it. Start slowly with an easy exercise such as walking, and then gradually build up your stamina by increasing your walking distance as your fatigue lessens. Maintain a good balance between mild exercise and periods of rest.

- Plan special or important activities when you know your strength will be at its highest level.

Sexual activity should take place when fatigue is at a minimum. Be open with your sexual partner about your level of fatigue. Skipping intercourse or just focusing on cuddling and kissing may be all that you feel comfortable with right now. Understand and accept your limits.

- Yoga, meditation, mindfulness training, and Tai Chi are all very good choices to help your brain and body relax.

- Listen to your favorite soothing music before bedtime, and avoid excessive stimulating activities before naps and bedtime. Quiet classical music can calm your brain and decrease disorganized thought patterns.

- If you are feeling anxious or depressed, ask for professional help. Peer support groups are located all over North America (contact the American Cancer Society).

- Spiritual and religious connections can soothe and uplift the human spirit. Talk with someone in your religious institution. Reading books about your faith, watching spiritually enlightening movies, and attending classes or discussion groups, or spending time with others in your spiritual circle may be helpful.

- Rest frequently when you are tired. Recognize your limits, and do not embarrassed to rest when necessary.

Consider using a cane, walker, wheelchair, or scooter if mobility is an issue. Use grab bars in bathrooms. Sit when getting dressed or putting on makeup, or allow yourself to hold onto the arm of your spouse, family member, or friend to keep steady while walking.

Excellent information about managing fatigue is available on the Internet. Contact the Oncology Nursing Society (*www.cancersymptoms.org*) or the National Comprehensive Cancer Network (*www.nccn.org*) for more information.

Improving Sleep Patterns

According to the National Commission on Sleep Disorders Research, over 40 million Americans suffer from some type of sleep disturbance—**insomnia** (inability to fall and remain asleep throughout the night), **sleep apnea** (stopping breathing during sleep leading to poor quality of sleep and not feeling refreshed in the

Insomnia
Disorder with sleep—inability to fall asleep.

Sleep apnea
A sleep disorder characterized by pauses in breathing during sleep.

59

Narcolepsy

A sleep disorder characterized by sudden and uncontrollable episodes of deep sleep.

Hypersomnia

A sleep disorder characterized by excessive amounts of sleepiness.

Restless leg syndrome

A condition that is characterized by an irresistible urge to move one's body or legs to stop uncomfortable or odd sensations.

morning), **narcolepsy** (immediate and unprovoked falling asleep), **hypersomnia** (sleeping too much), or **restless leg syndrome**. Many women report increased insomnia, sleep apnea, and poor sleep patterns immediately before or during the menopause transition. Hot flashes and other underlying illnesses may be significant contributors to poor sleep quality. Most people are chronically fatigued because we rarely allow ourselves sufficient rest for our bodies and minds to recover from our busy daily activities. Overwork and overscheduling, combined with poor sleep habits, cause a life of exhaustion.

Sleeping well at night can help you feel better and awake refreshed and may boost your energy level. If you have trouble sleeping or a poor quality of your sleep, try these suggestions at night:

- Go to bed and get up at the same time each day. Establish and stick with a nightly routine. Your body needs predictability.
- Keep the temperature in your bedroom comfortable. Hot flashes can interrupt sleep even if they do not awaken you during the night.
- Keep the bedroom quiet and dark when you are sleeping. Try earplugs or background or "white" noise such as a CD with ocean sounds or raindrops. If you cannot make your bedroom dark, wear a sleep mask. Unplug your telephone, cellular phone, or iPhone, and shut down your computer and BlackBerry.
- Do not let pets sleep in your bedroom. They are often "bed hogs" and can move around, thereby interrupting your sleep. If you want your pet nearby, then consider a special bed at the foot of your bed or somewhere else in the master bedroom!

- Create a bedtime routine. Play cards, read, or enjoy other quiet activities immediately before you go to bed. Most sleep experts suggest that you not watch television or use the Internet before bed, as these activities may be too stimulating.

- Use your bed only for sleep and sex. Create a loving, tranquil environment. Purchase new, comfortable sheets and linens. Try a nice feathery pillow cover!

- Take only your own prescription medications, and use them as directed. Take any prescribed sleeping pills 40 to 60 minutes before bedtime. Some fast-acting medications must be taken right before going into bed. Consult with your healthcare professional if you think that you may need a prescription sleep aid.

- Use a relaxation exercise just before going to sleep. Try muscle relaxation (while lying face up, tense and relax each muscle from the bottom of your feet to the top of your head), mental imagery, massage, a warm bath, calm music or a soothing classical symphony, or light reading.

- Do not eat a heavy or high-fat meal before going to bed. Limit your fluids before going to bed.

- Avoid caffeinated beverages, nicotine, and alcohol in the late afternoon and evening. Try drinking decaffeinated herbal teas that are calming (e.g., passionflower or chamomile).

- If you cannot fall asleep within a reasonable time, get out of bed and do something relaxing. Continue reading your book or listening to music. Staying in bed can become frustrating.

- Try keeping a sleep diary, including the time you go to bed, what you did before sleeping, when you took naps, and whether you wake up during the night.

TREATMENTS

Document how you feel in the morning, and bring this booklet to your healthcare provider, who may use this information to diagnosis a sleep disorder.

- If you cannot get your mind away from worries, make a list of your concerns and things you can do to decrease or eliminate that worry (e.g., ask the doctor about a symptom, discuss your fears with a friend or your partner). Organize your calendar for the next day. Sometimes just writing things in an organized fashion can be helpful. Then you can release your inner demand that they must be done immediately and understand that you will do them tomorrow, next week, or whenever.

Sometimes just writing things in an organized fashion can be helpful.

If you have trouble sleeping or a poor quality of your sleep, try these suggestions during the day:

- Exercise (any type each day, but not before bedtime).
- Keep a sleep diary to share with your doctor. Your healthcare clinician may be able to offer suggestions or prescribe a sleep aid.
- Do not take daytime naps.

Magnolia Myrick:

I think if you had "inner spiritual meaning" before cancer, then you will have it after, and maybe more so. I certainly did. If you didn't have it, the occasion of cancer is a real good time to search for meaning and truth, whatever that might mean to you, if for no other reason than it will make you feel better. Ask around if you think finding "inner spiritual meaning" or a connection to something or someone higher or greater than yourself will help. You'll find somewhere to start; go from there.

36. I am too stressed for sex. How can I manage my stress better?

Stress management is a learned skill. Although much stress is out of your control, how you organize yourself to respond to stress will directly relate to your quality of life. Stress can change your hormones and ultimately your sexual response. Women who suffer from severe and chronic stress often complain of decreased sexual interest. They may be uninterested in sex and often shun advances from their partners. The following suggestions offer methods you can use to manage your time and thought processes:

- *Revise your thinking.* Acknowledge frustration. Accept the things you cannot change. Forgive. Consider whether there might be more positive solutions to the problem. Take a break when needed. Sometimes the solution is staring you in the face—you might need only a short cooling period to discover the best action. Start at one place, and try to do what you can. Know your limits.

- *Choose a healthy diet and exercise regimen.* Following a diet rich in fruits, grains, and vegetables while decreasing saturated fats tends to lower your blood pressure. Limit caffeinated drinks because they can increase anxiety and cause rapid heart rates. Choose healthy, low-calorie snack foods. Your energy will return after eating a nutritious diet. Eat a diet that is rich in antioxidants, including strawberries, blueberries, and raspberries. Juice plus, a food supplement of fruits and vegetables, can help to energize the immune system. Preliminary research shows that women (and men and children) on Juice plus have increased levels of antioxidants, which can fight **free radicals**. Those

Free radicals

An atom or group of atoms that has at least one unpaired electron and is therefore unstable and highly reactive. It typically can cause damage to normal cells.

who take Juice plus often tell of decreased fatigue, boosted immunity, and overall health and wellness. It is food and many women and men swear by its effectiveness. It has anti-inflammatory properties and is widely researched in many prominent universities. Exercise away your stress. Often a brisk walk or a session at the gym will help clear your mind so that you can reframe your problems more creatively and manageably.

- *Plan.* Stay focused and organized. If you plan your day in advance, you are more likely to spend your time efficiently. Be sure to leave work at your designated time, delegate chores to family members (including children), or (if financially possible) hire extra housecleaning help. Your spouse or partner can always pitch in to get the dry cleaning, shop for food, or help the children do their homework. Divide and conquer household tasks.

- *Know and set your limits.* Is it really crucial that your bed be made every day? Is it okay to have some clothes on the floor once in a while? Choose not to get overly stressed if your home is not clean. Make active decisions to delay certain chores.

- *Say no!* Overextending yourself leads to increased stress and anxiety. Learning to say no, at appropriate times, to personal, social, or employment commitments is crucial. Be polite, yet firm, in your convictions. By saying no to certain projects, you remain focused on the activities that are most important. With practice, learning to say no becomes increasingly easier. You cannot be everything for everyone.

- *Relaxation techniques.* Meditation, yoga, or other relaxation techniques provide useful tools to help maintain an active lifestyle with a sense of tranquility. Stretching and Tai Chi classes are often offered inexpensively at your neighborhood YMCA or recreation center. Practice deep breathing for 5 to 10 minutes at a time (see Question 31). Try to clear your mind of all thoughts and concerns and just focus on your breath. Relax your muscles as you inhale and exhale, while letting your mind go completely blank. This exercise is a great stress buster early in the morning or late at night.

Many other therapeutic strategies are available. Professional counseling with a trained social worker, psychologist, or psychiatrist may help you work through unresolved childhood issues. Emotional patterns and responses to serious life events can emerge from the subconscious to the fully conscious adult in a safe way for healing. Getting a perspective from a professional therapist often opens new avenues of thinking about your situation. They specialize in helping you to develop coping strategies tailored to meet your emotional needs.

Magnolia Myrick:

Breathing, focusing on the breath, is as simple a form of meditation as there is, and as effective. Everything I read and hear about meditation says it is good and good for you. What do you have to lose? I have meditated off and on since college, but I do it regularly now, and without fail. It is a little effort with a big benefit. Wayne Dyer's Getting in the Gap *is a good, easy, and short how-to on meditating, but there are lots of books out there on meditation. Transcendental meditation is also an excellent and easy method learned in several hours of formal instruction, for which there is a fee. For more information, transcendental medication's nonprofit organization has a very good website. It is the first kind of meditation I learned and a fool-proof technique I can practice anytime, anywhere.*

37. How do Tamoxifen (AstraZeneca) and aromatase inhibitors affect sexual function?

Tamoxifen, manufactured by AstraZeneca, is a selective estrogen receptor modulator (SERM) that is often used to treat breast cancer and can exacerbate menopausal symptoms. SERMs have been linked with vaginal dryness, vaginal discharge, vaginal tenderness, changes in orgasm, and diminished libido. Studies examining the effects of Tamoxifen on sexual functioning in women are conflicting and inconclusive. The Breast Cancer Prevention Trial states that minor differences in sexual functioning were observed in Tamoxifen users. In contrast, Mortimer's study demonstrated no changes in any phase of female sexual response cycle for women who were taking Tamoxifen.

Femara (**Letrozole**) (Novartis oncology), Arimidex Anastrozole (AstraZeneca), and Aromasin Exemestane (Pfizer Pharmacology) are all **aromatase inhibitors**. These medications work by blocking the conversion of **testosterone** to estrogen and significantly lowering the levels of circulating estradiol. Although this action is often the objective of breast cancer therapy, they can aggravate menopausal symptoms and cause **osteopenia, osteoporosis, arthralgia**, decreased vaginal lubrication, vaginal dryness, and painful intercourse. Many women even discontinue their medications because of distressing and troublesome vaginal dryness and painful sex. More scientific trials are needed to address the sexual ramifications of these drugs. Many of the pharmaceutical companies are now becoming more actively involved in survivorship concerns, and sexuality is high on their radar screens. Survivorship initiatives are underway to help mitigate side effects while effectively managing the disease state.

38. My depression medication is hurting my sex drive. I feel sad and am crying a lot. How can I get a handle on my depression?

Throughout your journey with cancer, it is normal to feel anxious or depressed, as you may believe that you have lost a vital part of yourself and are worried about the future. When sadness persists and is combined with feelings of helplessness or hopelessness, a loss of or increased appetite, and sleep disturbances, a diagnosis of major depression may be considered. When your emotions interfere with your life, you are careless of your hygiene, you lack a zest for life, or you withdraw from social and professional commitments, it is time to seek professional help. If you find yourself making plans to hurt yourself or even think about ending your life, seek *immediate* medical attention. Today, depression is not seen as a sign of weakness or stigma—rather, it is a known and accepted neurobiological condition. Depression can be treated effectively with both medications and psychotherapy. Often, successful management might include a prescription of antidepressant medications combined with psychotherapy. The cause(s) of a major depression is often multifaceted, and thus, a multidimensional approach is required for effective treatment. Biological, psychological, and social factors are often addressed during therapy sessions. Individual counseling therapy involves visiting with a therapist alone. Group therapy is when a small number of people meet with a therapist together. Because some women find comfort in talking with other women who have undergone the same treatments or suffer from the same type of cancer, group therapy may be helpful. Cognitive behavioral therapy, interpersonal therapy, supportive psychotherapy, and psychodynamic psychotherapy are different programs that you may consider when

Today, depression is not seen as a sign of weakness or stigma—rather, it is a known and accepted neurobiological condition.

TREATMENTS

talking with your therapist(s). Many national cancer centers have posttreatment resource centers or survivorship programs that organize group support programs for both men and women, and sometimes they are cancer diagnosis specific. Other program events can include discussions about depression, sexual health, or other survivorship issues. Sharing your concerns and fears with others may be a way to help you regain control over your emotions.

Antidepressant medications can cause sexual side effects. The serotonin retake inhibitors often affect sexual interest, libido, or orgasm. An orgasm maybe less intense or the time to orgasm may be affected by your antidepressant medication. If you are having sexual side effects from your depression medication, discuss your concerns with your sexual healthcare provider. Sometimes switching medications can be helpful. Reassess whether you actually need to take the medication. Others plan sexual play when medications may be least offensive. If you take medications in the morning, plan sexual play in the morning before your next dose. In some recent studies, the addition a **PDE5 inhibitor** taken before sexual activity has been shown to be helpful for reversing or lessening serotonin retake inhibitor-induced sexual side effects. Before trying an antidote or switching your medications, consult with your healthcare team.

PDE5 inhibitor

Class of drugs which cause smooth muscle relaxation. Typically used in men and have been used effectively for the treatment of erectile difficulties.

39. What about pain medications? Do they affect sexual function?

Living in chronic pain can negatively affect your activities, and overall mental, physical, and emotional well-being are impacted. By controlling discomfort, you can effectively regain control of your life, enjoy a more active vibrant lifestyle, and enjoy social connections. Letting your pain get out of control often leads to feelings of anger, frustration, depression, or even isolation and stress.

Your oncology doctors, nurses, pharmacists, anesthesiologists, neurologists, and perhaps a specialist in pain management all help to manage pain. There is no reasonable rationale to suffer in silence, be stoic or brave, believe that discussing your pain or discomfort is a sign of weakness, or to even rationalize your suffering as being part of the healing process. Discuss your concerns with your healthcare team. Some patients who fail to discuss pain control mistakenly believe that if they do take prescribed pain medications they will become addicted. This is rarely the case, even if you are taking strong medications like narcotics or opioids. Some people fear the potential side effects, like constipation, nausea and vomiting, lightheadedness, feeling confused, or even a feeling of loss of control. Discuss your personal concerns with your doctor so that your dosing schedule can be modified or medications changed to minimize side effects while maximizing pain control.

There are many types of cancer pain, including acute, chronic, and breakthrough pain. Pain can come from the cancer tumor itself or be a result of the surgery, chemotherapy, or radiation therapy you have received. Phantom pain can occur at the site of an amputation or limb removal, and some women who have had mastectomies or complete breast removal can feel abnormal pain, sensations, or discomfort at the area where the breast is missing.

Sometimes cancer pain treatment will involve medications and nonmedical techniques that can minimize your pain. It may be helpful to develop and implement an adequate pain management plan with your healthcare team.

TREATMENTS

Some pain medication is over the counter, and others are prescribed by your doctor. Before your medical visit, write and bring a list all of the medications you are taking. These drugs can be analyzed so that possible side effects or drug interactions can be minimized. Some of the medications typically used for pain control are listed here. This list is not exhaustive, and new medications may be offered by your doctor. Pain medications can come in the form of pills (taken by mouth), patches, and liquids (elixir), or they may be injected into your bloodstream (intravenous), muscle (intramuscular), or the space around nerve endings in your spine (epidural). Suppositories also may be used (see Question 27).

Magnolia Myrick said:

I'm one of those people who "hates to take things" like pain or sleep medications. And that is ridiculous. I've finally come to realize I want my body's energy to heal *and not to struggle with pain or insomnia. I know when I need them and when I don't, and so will you. I think of these medicines as working with my body, and that's what we want.*

40. How can I control pain and still have sex?

If you are in pain, sexual activity may not be important to you. Many pain medications can change hormones and thus affect sexual appetite and interest. Discuss your pain medication selections with your provider. Plan sexual activity when your pain is at a minimum. Let your partner know that you are in pain and would prefer to snuggle rather than have intercourse. Some sexual medicine specialists will actually advocate use of pain medications before sexual activity. Finding a comfortable sexual position may also limit pain. Sometimes stretching exercises or even guided imagery can be helpful. Try to control your level of pain with both Eastern and Western methods of pain management.

As with any surgery, one should expect pain—the amount of pain experienced is usually dependent on the extent of surgery. Breast surgery is no different. Breast-saving surgery, for example, creates less pain than a mastectomy. Mastectomy alone may create less pain than a mastectomy with reconstruction. However, every woman and her experience with are unique. Surprisingly, lymph node sampling creates the greatest amount of pain and also causes range of motion issues. Physical therapy may be helpful in some cases.

Touching and massaging may help reduce some of the painful areas and create a sense of closeness and intimacy. Gently rubbing the scar area helps to reduce formation of scar tissue. After the surgical line is healed, lotion or oil can be used. If a partner is involved, this can be seen as very loving and caring. Some of the medications taken during treatment create severe bone pain in the long bones and the small of the back. This pain also can be reduced by gently rubbing, possibly with an oil or lotion.

Neuropathy, a result of medications, is usually experienced in the hands and/or feet. Rubbing these areas helps to reduce the pain and create intimacy. Estrogen deprivation can cause the wall of the vagina to thin and make intercourse painful. This is a time for creativity so that sexual activities can be meaningful but still not include penetration.

Neuropathy
Damage to nerves of the peripheral nervous system.

41. What are bioidentical hormones? Are they safe?

According to the American College of Obstetricians and Gynecologists committee, compounded bioidentical hormones are created, mixed, and packaged by a pharmacist who can customize the product according to the physician's specifications. All **bioidentical hormones** are synthetically created. Your body makes a form of estrogen called estradiol, and bioidentical estrogen is estradiol. Estrace Cream contains bioidentical estradiol, or the same estrogen within your body, and is pharmaceutically created by Warner Chicott Pharmaceuticals. Pharmaceutical products are tightly and strictly regulated by the governmental agencies for reliability, consistency, and purity.

Bioidentical hormones

Hormonal preparations that have a similar structure to humans' naturally occurring hormones.

Most compounded products have not undergone strict scientific study, and concerns about safety, purity, and efficacy may exist. When the compounding pharmacist mixes special hormonal blends, he or she uses bioidentical hormones. In actuality, Premarin is the one all-natural hormone. It is derived from horse urine.

Compounded products have the same risks as conventional pharmacologically produced hormones. Also, no medically recognized governing organization like the FDA officially regulates compounding substances; there is often lack of consistency, purity, and reproducibility. Thus, many women on compounded hormones complain of erratic hormonal fluctuations.

The most common compounded hormones include dehydroepiandrosterone, pregnenolone, testosterone, progesterone, estrone, estradiol, and estriol. They are administered in the following ways: oral, sublingual, implants, injectables, or suppositories. Biest consists of 20% estradiol and 80% estriol. Another, Triest, contains 10% estradiol, 10% estrone, and 80% estriol. Most insurance companies will not reimburse for these compounded products, and thus, they can be expensive for the individual. Many do not contain the same amount of concentrated active ingredients claimed on their packaging. No scientific data support the claim that bioidentical hormones are safer than conventional prescribed hormonal therapy.

Those who use compounded bioidentical hormones often advocate for salivary oral testing of hormones. Some claim that the salivary hormone results can be used to tailor an individual preparation for a woman and her unique hormonal needs. Unfortunately, there is no medical evidence that salivary hormones provide any clinically useful information. Salivary hormones depend on a multitude of factors, including the hormone tested and the time of day the test was conducted. Also, there may not be a direct correlation between salivary hormones and biologically active hormone levels, clinical state, or therapeutic results. A large variation of levels exists within the same individual and between individuals. If you are considering taking bioidentical hormones or are now taking a prescribed compound, know that it may be dangerous. Discuss the risks of bioidentical hormones with your cancer specialist.

Systemic treatment with hormones either compounded or pharmaceutically created is not the mainstay of treatment for women with hormonally sensitive tumors like breast cancer. Some providers will treat their patients with these products, but treatment remains highly controversial. Because tumor reoccurrence is possible, even if your first tumor is estrogen and progesterone receptor negative, your oncological team may not feel comfortable with hormones; however, the situation is different with minimally absorbed local vaginal estrogen products.

42. My range of motion has been affected by lymphedema. What can I do?

Most patients experience a limited range of motion in the arm from which lymph nodes were removed. Discomfort in the **axilla region**, down the back side of the arm and sometimes generating down into the entire arm, is often resolved after healing takes place but still sometimes persists. Lymphedema, a chronic condition that can be treated but not cured, occurs when lymph in the arm is unable to go back into the body to be dissolved. It creates swelling, pain, and discomfort. The arm with lymphedema may appear larger than the other. Approximately 30% of breast cancer patients who have undergone lymph node removal will get lymphedema. Some lymphedema is mild and can be managed with manual and physical therapy, but some cases are severe and cause considerable pain for the patient. In severe cases, the arm, and sometimes the hand, becomes large, swollen, and painful. Women may be unable to wear clothes with tight sleeves. They must wear a heavy bandage on their arm and a heavy glove on their hand. The bandages may be unattractive, making the individual feel unattractive. Although some spouses are supportive by providing bandaging and care, the lymphema may still present a deterrent to feelings of sexuality and sensuality and can interfere with lovemaking.

A new and exciting organization, called Lymphediva (*www.lymphedivas.com*), makes specially designed compression sleeves from colorful, sexy, and comfortable material. They offer interesting fashionable prints from wild

Axilla region

Armpit, underarm, or oxte.

leopard skin to bright fuchsia and paisley. Lymphediva is a family-owned company that is run by parents whose daughter died of breast cancer; their mission is to enrich the lives of breast cancer survivors, to add to their quality of life, and to help improve their sexual self-esteem.

43. What about breast cancer sexuality for the single woman or parent?

Being a single parent combined with a breast cancer diagnosis makes for a very difficult situation. Concerns include child care, transportation, and helping the child to feel safe. If the children are teenagers, there may be issues of unmet expectations. Teens need their mothers, but their mothers may be occupied with treatment and recovery.

If you are in a new relationship, you may receive added care and support; however, if your new partner is overwhelmed, you may feel alone. With so much uncertainty in your life, you may be unable to devote the time, energy, and attention to a relationship. Despite this, some woman meet a new partner while undergoing chemotherapy and enjoy a long-lasting relationship.

If you have small children in your home, they are going to need their mother's attention and time. They may be afraid of your illness, your inability to take care of them, your return to the hospital, or death.

If you are not in a serious relationship, dating may need to be put on hold until you complete treatment and are feeling healthy. Single women may be concerned about disclosure. When do you tell a new love interest that you have had or will have a mastectomy or that you may not be capable of having children? This is a personal decision.

Clearly, the issues of bodily changes should not be disclosed immediately before going into a sexual act with your new partner. Remember that not all partners will be supportive. It is good get mentally prepared for several different reactions, one of which may be rejection.

Magnolia Myrick:

So there I was: a groovy single chick with an active social life in New York City—with breast cancer, which is very not groovy. I just decided I would hold my head high, wig and all, and keep myself out there in the dating world as much as I felt up to it. I usually waited until I'd gotten to know him a bit to talk about the cancer. And if it never got that far then, it wasn't an issue anyway. If he ended the relationship because he was put off by the cancer, then he's got integrity issues, and I don't want him anyway. I hate to say that I do believe this happened a couple of times (and one of them was a doctor). But listen, this is the kind of thing I want to know about someone sooner rather than later. Anyone can be a fair-weather friend. I want the through-thick-and-thin kind of friend, and so do you.

In retrospect, it probably would have been easier to skip dating while I was in treatment, but it would have been such a lifestyle change for me that it might have made me more self-conscious than I already was. It's not a straightforward issue, and your decision would depend on what your existing social life is like and what you want it to be during treatment. And hey, taking it one day at a time is always a good decision.

If you're in a relationship, the question becomes what if we stay together, or marry, and the cancer comes back? We have to talk about this. He could be in the position of becoming my caretaker. It's a big deal. It's also worth pointing out that he might get cancer, or be hit by a bus, and that I might become his caretaker. They don't put that line in there about "in sickness or in health" for nothing. I'm not a therapist, but it seems to me you need to figure this out about anyone you are seriously involved with. And if you don't like what you've figured out, bye–bye birdie.

44. What about women in same–sex relationships?

Same sex-relationships face many of the same stressors as heterosexual relationships. If the relationship is "solid" emotionally before a breast cancer diagnosis, it will persist after the treatment and recovery process. Conversely, unstable relationships may falter and even end under the turmoil of diagnosis and treatment. A same-sex relationship may be more empathetic, particularly with reference to understanding the meaning of the loss of a breast.

Women who love and are sexual with other women have significant concerns about changes in the breast tissue. Address sexual concerns and how breast cancer and its therapy may affect sexual function. Lesbian sexuality has often been neglected in the medical publications and in the media. Approximately 3% to 5% of the female population is comprised of self-identified lesbians who enjoy sexual relationships with partners. Many are in long-term committed relationships that share social, financial, and child-rearing responsibilities.

According to the Lesbian Health Fund's founder, Kate O'Hanlan, who is also a former president of the Gay and Lesbian Medical Association, there are many health care concerns that may negatively impact a healthy sexual life that lesbians should discuss with their healthcare providers. Some of these are shared with the general

If the relationship is "solid" emotionally before a breast cancer diagnosis, it will persist after the treatment and recovery process.

female population, including risks for breast cancer (some women over the age of 40 do not get regular mammograms, do not perform self breast examinations or receive clinical breast examinations), gynecological health care, osteoporosis, and domestic violence. Of particular concern to lesbians, issues related to depression, anxiety, and other psychiatric illnesses, due to possible chronic stress from **homophobia**, stress from disapproving family, and/or unfriendly work and social environments, are important to address. These issues can result in substance and alcohol abuse and excessive tobacco use. Obesity may also be a concern. Cardiovascular health care is critical and screenings for diabetes, high cholesterol, and high blood pressure should be done regularly, as well as improving overall diet and fitness.

Some medical illnesses or surgical procedures that impact the breasts may also adversely affect the sexual pleasure of lesbians who focus on breast caressing and stimulation for a large part of their sexual arousal. Those who have had surgical alteration or removal of this erotic area of their body may feel saddened by the loss of this sexual organ. Clitoral arousal and stimulation may also be impacted by medications that blunt arousal (depressive medications). "Lesbian bed death" is a term that sex researcher Pepper Schwartz coined to describe diminished sexual passion or sexual activity in any long-term relationship, may also be a concern.

Homophobia

Range of negative attitudes and feelings towards homosexuality and people identified as gay or lesbian.

PART THREE

Psychosocial Issues

What are common psychosexual problems
that couples experience?

What is sexual self-esteem?

What body image issues might a woman
with breast cancer experience?

More . . .

45. What are common psychosexual problems that couples experience?

Many couples fall into a pattern of sexual activity that is not satisfying to one or both partners and do not know how to make necessary changes. A breast cancer diagnosis may be the catalyst that allows discussion and experimentation to take place. Our culture stresses female breasts as an important part of sexuality and femininity; thus, losing a breast or both breasts to cancer can affect your sense of value. Women who were confident about their sexual attractiveness before breast surgery may feel insecure afterward. If breast and nipple sensitivity increases a woman's sexual pleasure, she will experience a loss when it is gone. Although the skin will again become somewhat sensitive, rarely is the sensitivity the same as it was before surgery. A woman's breasts do not define who she is as a woman or a sexual partner.

Not all women choose to have reconstruction after surgery; however, sometimes women find a lot of sensitivity from their scar and derive sexual pleasure from this. Some may feel guilty about this new-found pleasure. Others experience pain and discomfort after surgery that do not resolve; thus, the breast area no longer provides sexual pleasure. Partners often report that the reconstructed breast is just as sensual as a normal breast.

Many other factors besides a breast cancer diagnosis could affect a woman's satisfactory sexual life. **Cardiovascular disease, atherosclerosis, hypertension**, and **diabetes** may negatively impact healthy sexuality. In woman, diabetes has been shown to lessen desire, arousal, lubrication, and orgasm, which damages nerves in the clitoris and penis, literally stunting the ability to experience sensuality. Other factors like aches and pains

Cardiovascular disease

The class of diseases that involve the heart or blood vessels (arteries and veins).

Atherosclerosis

A condition in which fatty material collects along the walls of arteries.

Hypertension

High blood pressure; an abnormality in arterial blood pressure that typically results from a thickening of the blood vessel wall. It is a risk factor for many illnesses, including heart attacks, heart failure, and stroke, or end-stage kidney disease.

Diabetes

a medical disease characterized with abnormal sugar metabolism and levels.

associated with aging or sleep disorders decrease sexual desire and performance. Obesity is also associated with lack of enjoyment of sexual activity, lack of sexual desire, difficulties with sexual performance, and avoidance of sexual encounters.

Smoking, alcohol, drug abuse, stress, and side effects from almost any medication, particularly antidepressants, can impact sexual arousal and response at any age. Significant psychological factors that affect loss of sexuality include perceived unattractiveness. Sexuality in humans is made of desire, arousal, orgasm, and resolution. Each phase is governed by corresponding brain chemicals, along with contributing hormonal influences. When the brain is experiencing a chemical deficiency in any of the four primary areas, the desire for sex diminishes.

Significant psychological factors that affect loss of sexuality include perceived unattractiveness.

46. What is sexual self-esteem?

How you view yourself as a sexual person is often defined as sexual self-esteem. If you have a positive sexual self-esteem, then you have embraced your sexual identity, think of yourself as sexy, and are embracing your body as it has changed with age and disease. In contrast, those with negative sexual self-esteem feel unattractive, not sexy, and often ashamed of their bodies and how they perform sexually.

When you are bald and nauseated from cancer treatments, sensuality and sexuality may not be important, but intimacy may be on your mind. You may need reassurance about your sexuality and desirability. Ask your partner for what you need in order to get reassurance. If you do not have someone in your life, find other ways to make sure that your sexual self-esteem is intact. Most women are comfortable with their degree of femininity, but many women are unsure of themselves regarding sexuality and their roles with regard to pleasure and pleasing.

47. What body image issues might a woman with breast cancer experience?

Women may see themselves as too fat, too tall, too short. They are bombarded in the media with the perfect body, perfect face, and perfect hair and are told what they must do to achieve perfection. Plastic surgery is rampant, as is dieting, exercising, and women's focus on their outward physical appearance.

If you do not feel attractive before your diagnosis, you may have lowered self-esteem after treatment or diagnosis. Certainly, having one breast or no breasts at all affects your self-image and feelings of adequacy.

In our culture, breasts define who we are as wives, lovers, and mothers. A bare breast, or a hint of a bare breast, has immediate sexual inferences or indications. Thus, the loss or a change in the shape or sensation of a breast often has a significant impact on self-esteem. Our culture is enamored with youth, and unfortunately, aging affects all parts of the body linked with sexual function, both internally and externally. With a breast cancer diagnosis, you may have a woman who has great difficulty seeing herself as desirable.

48. *What are sensuality, intimacy, and love?*

Both men and women confuse lust with love, sexuality with the sex act, sensuality with appeal, and intimacy with sexuality. This confusion can lead to a misunderstanding about how relationships change and mature over time.

Being "in love" is depicted in the media as a time of high lust, when couples cannot stand to be apart from each other. Love often signifies a joining as one in your life journey. Lust is often perceived as carnal drive that lessens with the length of the relationship. As this lust lessens, sometimes you may falsely think that you are "falling out of love." However, a relationship may progress from erotic sexual lust to the deep commitment of lasting love. Irrespective of which phase of "love" one is in, when you are dealing with cancer diagnosis and treatment, it is important to feel desired. Feelings of desirability are also linked to preference. What do I think is sexy? What about when I dress a certain way? Walk a certain way? Speak in a certain tone?

Take some time to explore the notions of love, sex, intimacy with and without your partner. You will be surprised at your differing or similar perspectives. This is an exercise in communication, and you will be closer to your own sexual self and that of your partner.

49. *What is loss of sexual interest in intimacy or sex?*

Cancer may cause much of the loss of interest in intimacy for women. Those who had active breast caressing as part of their sexual repertoire will mourn the loss of this activity, leading to feelings of loss, ultimately demonstrating clinically as lowered sexual desire. Chemotherapy causes both nausea and fatigue and affects a woman's sexual hormone levels, such as estrogen, progesterone, and testosterone, all factors that reduce feelings of desire. Some of the medications discussed earlier to help keep disease stable can also have effects on the sexual response cycle, including desire.

Hypoactive sexual desire disorder (HSSD)

Lowered sexual interest that is often characterized by absence of sexual thoughts and fantasies—it is associated with distress.

The emotional impact of the diagnosis alone causes many women to experience anxiety and depression. Many women suffer from **hypoactive sexual desire disorder (HSSD)**. New exciting scientific developments are underway for possible treatments for women who are suffering with this condition.

Often, in the face of treatment, sexual wellness is not a priority. Nurture yourself. Take an adult time out! Spend quality time alone; it will make you a better mother, wife, and daughter. Set limits, and make yourself and your relationship, sensuality, and sexuality a priority.

In our busy lives, we let our jobs and careers and family obligations interfere with our need for intimacy. Quick sexual encounters may be exciting and satisfying, but there is also the need for reaffirmation that you are loved intensely. Deeper intimacy and emotional connection can be built when time and energy are present and you make yourself and your partner a priority.

Sexual health has been linked to overall health. Focus on your intimate partnerships. Love, sex, and intimacy will help you heal and recover from the devastation of cancer.

Sexual health has been linked to overall health. Focus on your intimate partnerships.

50. What is psychosexual counseling?

Concerns about sexuality and intimacy are very private matters, but you may need professional counseling in this area, both before and after a breast cancer diagnosis. Many healthcare providers are reluctant and uncomfortable to enter into these discussions. Sometimes the provider will need you to broach the topic, and if you feel discounted, do not get discouraged! Think about seeking those who are sensitive to your sexual wellness concerns.

Psychosexual counseling can help a woman understand that beauty truly comes from within and that losing a breast should not affect your self-image. It involves meeting with a therapist and talking about what is happening in your sexual life as a result of cancer. Be certain to ask about credentials and experience in dealing with breast cancer patients.

51. What is marital counseling?

Many spouses or partners feel very scared and confused during the process of a breast cancer diagnosis and treatment. The partner, lover, boyfriend, or spouse cannot do the surgery and often cannot help with the treatment. They often feel helpless and do not know what to do or say. They may experience a strong desire to take care of and protect the spouse, to be close and loving with their partner, but may be afraid to approach her sexually or intimately. Often, so much about their relationship changes in a short time. Partners often become caregivers and are suddenly 100% responsible for domestic duties and childcare during cancer treatment. Their role in the dyadic relationship may change dramatically. They often mean well but sometimes are confused about how to be supportive and encouraging without pressuring their partner.

The patient may deal with the physical and emotional impact of surgery, radiation, or chemotherapy. She may fear how her cancer will affect her relationships and may have feelings of not being the best mother or good wife and causing her family pain. She may even feel guilty that she now is unable to fulfill her duties as childcare giver, mother, housewife, and lover. She may also be upset about her inability to maintain social and employment commitments, thus directly impacting the family's financial well-being.

Little or no information is available to help couples and families get through this crisis. Sometimes couples function well with traditional sex roles (e.g., the wife attended to the children and home), but when roles change due to illness, the partner must now take on new responsibilities and may feel tremendously overwhelmed. Unconscious anger and resentment may build and need to be addressed. Sometimes other family members, mothers, mothers-in-law, or others, move into the family home to provide assistance, and this may increase marital strain. Privacy issues are also a consideration when outside caregivers are involved.

Counselors are trained to deal with a couple's marital conflict and issues. When cancer invades a marriage and relationship, you may need some assistance in reestablishing effective and loving communication styles. Sometimes you may need an impartial listener who can help guide you to a sense of relationship harmony. Seek professional psychological couples counseling if your relationship has suffered as a result of the breast cancer. Make sure that you and your partner are comfortable with the counselor's care. Sometimes medical insurances will cover or reimburse the fees for counseling; thus, always check your benefits with your medical insurance carrier.

52. *What is individual counseling?*

If married or in a relationship, you may be concerned about your partner dealing with the loss of your breast(s). If you are single, you may be concerned about how this may affect your ability to attract a partner. Individual counseling allows you to discuss these issues in a private setting.

A good place to discuss these concerns is with a therapist who knows your history. If not, ask your healthcare provider for a referral. The counselor should be sensitive to breast cancer issues. Do your homework by using the Internet to check their credentials and expertise.

A good counselor will be able to help you address your concerns for the future and help you develop a new strong sense of self and sensuality. He or she will also help you accept the new normal, possibly even a change of physical appearance, and will help you to cope with stress, depression, fear of cancer reoccurrence, and anger.

A good counselor will be able to help you address your concerns for the future and help you develop a new strong sense of self and sensuality.

53. What are some counseling techniques?

Many types of therapeutic approaches exist. If you have a real-time immediate crisis and want suggestions on how to solve a particular problem, you may want to choose a therapist who has experience in crisis management.

If you believe the way you are handling your diagnosis is the result of things that happened in your past, it might be helpful to work with a therapist who will examine your past. Sometimes negative thinking about a certain issue can be addressed in short-term cognitive behavior therapy, where negative thoughts are recognized replaced with more helpful functional thoughts and behaviors.

If your family or partner needs to be part of the therapeutic process, find a therapist who includes couples and family therapy. For resolving personal issues, find a therapist who will help you to integrate your past with your current situation and help to guide you to some understanding and resolution.

Some therapists have a practice that is focused on the patient who has experienced a cancer diagnosis. Others have expertise in sexuality and intimacy. Seek a therapist that will address your issues, and change therapists if your needs are not met. Some therapists can integrate a variety of differing approaches.

Some therapists practice cognitive behavioral therapy, which solves problems concerning emotions, behaviors, and thoughts through a goal-oriented and systematic procedure. Sometimes behaviors and thoughts need to be changed to help in the healing process.

Other therapists mainly may listen (talk therapy) and provide feedback and insight to the patient to correct abnormal thoughts or provide simple suggestions to change abnormal behavior. **Psychoanalytic therapy** and other forms of therapy may also offer some help for other patients.

Magnolia Myrick:

As a professional writer and editor, I'm in the business of creativity. As an amateur painter, avid cook, outdoors lover, and enthusiast of lots (probably too many) things, I'm in the business of creativity (and fun) in the off hours, too. This is not to trivialize all of the serious issues and responsibilities that life with cancer entails, but you don't have to think about them all the time. Doing something that gets you out of your head and into your heart and soul—something that brings you joy—is not just important but good for you. You hear me? Good for you. It can be a tiny thing: reading a poem, baking a cake, riding a bike. Or a big thing: writing a book, teaching a class, climbing Kilimanjaro. I go to the Church of Whatever Works, and anybody can join.

Psychoanalytic therapy

A body of ideas developed by Austrian physician Sigmund Freud and continued by others. It is primarily devoted to the study of human psychological functioning and behavior, the primary focus is to reveal the unconscious content of a client's psyche in an effort to aleviate psychic tension.

PSYCHOSOCIAL ISSUES

PART FOUR

Sexuality and Sexual Function After Breast Cancer

How can I explore my new sexuality
after breast cancer?

What is the difference between sexual performance
and sexual pleasure?

What specific sexual health management
therapies can I expect?

More . . .

54. How can I explore my new sexuality after breast cancer?

Some women may not look at having a breast cancer diagnosis as a completely negative experience—their diagnosis helped them to reprioritize their lives and became a liberating experience, particularly in the area of sexuality and intimacy. Because many aspects of body and function may be physically different, a cancer diagnosis is often viewed as an opportunity to experiment sexually. Some who have lost one breast focus their lovemaking on the remaining breast.

You may find that other erotic areas are actually more sensitive to touch and arousal than your breasts were; thus, your lovemaking may have taken on a much more expanded, exciting, and sexual dimension.

According to an ancient legend, Amazon women warriors would cut off their right breasts in order to use their bows and arrows more effectively. They were excellent, strong, magnificent fighters! If it is helpful, consider yourself a warrior. Some women have had their scars tattooed with trees and flowers and butterflies.

Sometimes the face of cancer allows you to step far out of your usual comfort zone. Sexually and personally explore your limits. Do not put off what you want to do!

55. What is the difference between sexual performance and sexual pleasure?

Many couples in our society remain goal oriented, and sex is considered a success only if there is penetration that is coupled with explosive orgasmic response. Nothing could be further from the truth! Often, the shifting of the ideal is important in sexual wellness. Focus on pleasure and enjoyment of the sexual experience. So what if there is no penetration, no orgasms, or a less-than-perfect **erection**? Togetherness and shared experience and connectedness are your ultimate goals.

Performance and pleasure do not go hand in hand. Focus on sexual togetherness rather than on the concept of penis in vagina or on orgasm. Very erotic noninsertive sexual play is also important. **Foreplay**—manual, oral, and digital stimulation—can be red-hot exciting for many couples, as can a steamy make-out session. Men and women should keep in mind that a "quickie" can be fun and emotionally exciting and very pleasurable. It is not always necessary to have a big romantic buildup to a sex encounter. Providing pleasure to a partner, even when you are not feeling particularly sexual, is part of caring for the needs of that partner.

If you are either physically or emotionally uncomfortable with a request of a partner, refuse or find another activity that is pleasing to both. Decide together what you want to include in your lovemaking sessions. Maybe you could experiment with oral sex or with a new type of sexual accessories?

Sexuality and intimacy do not always have to end in the sex act. Many activities are sexual, and many more are intimate. The more you and your partner experiment, the more opportunity there is to discover a vast treasure chest of sexual experiences and expression.

Erection

The expansion and hardening or stiffening of the sexual organ—it may be the penis, clitoris, or nipples—in response to sexual fantasy or stimulation.

Foreplay

Sexual behavior engaged in during the early part of the sexual encounter, with the aim of intensifying sexual arousal or pleasure.

56. How does aging affect sexual desire?

Unfortunately, with aging, for both men and women, comes a loss of sexual desire and decreased sexual performance. At 20 years old, a man may experience an erection daily or even more often; at 70, he may have only one weekly. For others, sexual response does not change with age.

In addition to a breast cancer diagnosis and treatment, other problems such as heart disease, hypertension, diabetes, menopause, kidney disease, and medications can affect sexual satisfaction, desire, and performance. Most people have at least one or two chronic medical illnesses as they age that will affect their sexual functioning.

At least 64% of Americans are obese, which can directly impact the sexual response in both men and women. Obese women can experience changes in arousal, vaginal lubrication, orgasm intensity, strength of orgasm, and overall sexual satisfaction.

External factors like smoking, alcohol and drug abuse, stress, fatigue and anxiety as well as the side effects from medication, particularly antihypertensive and antidepressants, can impact sexual arousal and response at any age.

External factors like smoking, alcohol and drug abuse, stress, fatigue and anxiety as well as the side effects from medication, particularly antihypertensive and antidepressants, can impact sexual arousal and response at any age. A person's perceived unattractiveness caused by aging can attribute to loss of sexuality. We all get older and carry a few more pounds and often are not aging gracefully. Sometimes we let ourselves go and head for the piece of cheese cake when we should be heading to the gym. Sometimes we take personal hygiene issues for granted. Have you neglected your personal hygiene or your weight? When was the last time you went to the hairdresser?

57. What changes in family dynamics can occur with breast cancer?

A women's entire family deals with the effects of breast cancer diagnosis. Partners who were used to being cared for now may become caregivers. If the woman has been working and contributing to the household income and is now not able to work, financial hardship may be present. All of these changes in the relationship may be played out in the bedroom. Underlying conflicts often can be boiled down to issues relating to power and control. Schedules, childcare, and chores need to be adjusted to accommodate treatment, recovery time, and doctors' appointments. Often, these changes are taken on willingly in the beginning of treatment but become burdensome as treatment progresses.

Even after the initial diagnosis and treatment, some women fear that their cancer will return; thus, they are reluctant to return to their normal lives, fearing that it may have been part of the cause of their disease.

Some may seek what they feel could be positive changes in their lives. Some get rid of the microwaves and processed food, whereas others become vegetarians and plant herb and vegetable gardens. A person may consider not returning to work or cutting back on some of the responsibilities. Another may quest for supplements and herbs. This may be difficult for other members of the family. The partner who is accustomed to "meat and potatoes" may be shocked when the traditional roast beef meal is replaced with tofu and salad greens.

Sometimes a woman "feels" the true emotional impact after treatment ends and she looks retrospectively at her "journey." Often, family members do not understand this, as they want this entire experience to be over. They will say, "But you're better now. Why would you want to go to a support group?" or "Why can't things be the way they were before your diagnosis?" It may make them feel unsafe when one dwells on the cancer diagnosis.

Cancer patients may take time for themselves that they had never done before. These changes can create great tension within the family. Be sure to focus on family meetings and improved communication! Discuss your concerns with your entire family, and allow time for feedback and discussion. Compromise is essential in solving conflict.

58. How does a sexual healthcare provider assess sexual functioning?

Some patients complain of having a low libido and changes in orgasm or arousal. Sexual pain disorders like **dyspareunia** (pain during intercourse) and **vaginismus** (reflexive contracture and tightening of the pelvic and vaginal muscles) are also prevalent. Discuss your sexual concerns with your healthcare providers. Specialists are available who focus on the oncological patient and sexual functioning.

Dyspareunia
Painful intercourse.

Vaginismus
An involuntary tightening of the vaginal muscles when the vagina is penetrated. The action can cause significant distress and pain.

A sexual healthcare provider will get a medical and gynecological history, a comprehensive general physical and genital examination, and a psychological as well as psychosexual examination. A complete medical and obstetrical history may provide some clues about the origin of the sexual complaint. Medications, including dose, time of day for administration, and possible side effects, will be discussed. Also, complementary and alternative therapies should also be discussed. Give your provider a list of prescription and over-the-counter medications you are taking, including supplements and vitamins.

Laboratory tests, such as a blood laboratory of various hormones or radiological evaluation, may be appropriate. Sometimes hormones or thyroid function is measured. Glucose and lipid function/cholesterol may also be assessed.

A sexual history will include sexual status, orientation, and past sexual experience; these concerns are important to discuss. Patients may also be encouraged to see a sexual medicine specialist/gynecologist and or a certified counselor or therapist for initial evaluations and follow-up.

Because sexual dysfunction is often complex and multidimensional, an individual's treatment may involve several different approaches. Healthy, satisfying sexual functioning and treatment success are impacted by a variety of factors, including medical illnesses, hormonal levels, relationship concerns, partner availability, underlying psychiatric disorders, general medical well-being, and cultural and religious behaviors.

59. Do many cancer survivors experience sexual complaints?

According to recent statistics from the American Cancer Society, with technological treatments and advancements in diagnostics and therapeutics, an estimated 60% of cancer survivors will live at least 5 years after their diagnosis. In 2009, over 11 million people were cancer survivors in the United States. Sexual complaints occur in up to 90% of women who have been diagnosed with cancer, and the number of women with posttreatment sexual dysfunction range from 30% to 100%. Unfortunately, these sexual complaints—lowered interest, vaginal discomfort, or pain—persist for many years, but are common and treatable conditions. There is no need to suffer in silence.

You are not alone if you have some sexual complaints. You may feel embarrassed or ashamed to discuss the issues with your healthcare providers. Nevertheless, your provider should be receptive to helping you with these deeply private issues. However, if your healthcare provider is uncomfortable or does not have the skills to deal with these sexual concerns, do not get discouraged. Do not give up! Review the Resources section starting on page 159 to help find another provider who can help answer all of your concerns, as this will ultimately enhance your quality of life.

You are not alone if you have some sexual complaints.

60. What specific sexual health management therapies can I expect?

Listed here are a variety of therapeutic options that the sexual medicine specialist may perform in order to treat your sexual complaints effectively.

Hypercholes-terolemia

The presence of an abnormal amount of cholesterol in the cells and plasma of the blood.

- *Treatment of systemic illnesses.* Cancer survivors often have other underlying medical conditions and illnesses that directly impact their sexual health. Evaluation and treatment of chronic illnesses, such as uncontrolled hypertension, **hypercholesterolemia**, and/or an underlying thyroid dysfunction, can be simple to identify. Arthritis or lymphedema from surgery or therapy may impact your finding comfortable sexual positions. Uncontrolled diabetes may influence veins, arteries, and nerves in the genital pelvic region, impacting blood flow and directly affect excitement.

Underlying genital infections like **candida** (yeast), bacterial **vaginitis**, and **trichomoniasis** should be effectively treated. Often, sexual specialists include screening, such as a complete blood profile, to rule out anemia, complete lipid profiles, glucose screening, and prolactin levels. Estrogen, testosterone, adrenal hormones, as well as progesterone and other hormonal profiles, are typically measured.

In the acute crisis of cancer care, pre-existing medical illnesses can sometimes be neglected. In long-term follow-up, however, treating any underlying chronic medical illnesses improves your general physical and mental well-being, as well as your sexuality.

- *Medications.* Most medications can affect the female sexual response cycle and cause sexual problems. Antidepressants and antihypertensive medications can change sexual desire, arousal, and orgasm. Ask your healthcare provider to check pharmacologic guides to identify potential offending agents and consider substituting another less offensive drug. Sexual pharmacology textbooks and the Internet provide a quick reference (be sure to review the National Institutes of Health and respected medical school web sites; see the Resources section on page 159). Some over-the-counter medications—like allergy medicines—can cause or exacerbate vaginal dryness. The medical treatment of sexual dysfunction often includes changing medication regimens, altering dosing and/or time intervals, or switching to a new drug. You should never abruptly stop any prescribed medication without first consulting with your prescribing provider. Some recent medical studies show that women who suffer from sexual dysfunction as a result of their antidepressant medications (like serotonin reuptake inhibitors) may benefit from **phosphodiesterase inhibitors** such as Viagra

Candida

Yeast infection typically occurs in the vagina and can be associated with itchiness and vaginal discharge.

Vaginitis

Inflammation of the vagina.

Trichomoniasis

A common sexually transmitted disease caused by the parasite Trichomonas vaginalis and infecting the urinary tract or vagina.

Phosphodiesterase inhibitors

Drugs that block one or more of the five subtypes of the enzyme phosphodiesterase (PDE), therefore preventing the inactivation of the intracellular second messengers cyclic adenosine monophosphate (cAMP) and cyclic guanosine monophosphate (cGMP) by the respective PDE subtype(s).

A well-balanced, nutritious diet combined with an active aerobic exercise plan is vital.

Sildenafil (Pfizer), Cialis Tadalafil (Lilly ICOS), or Levitra (Vardenafil) (Bayer Pharmaceutical and GlaxoSmithKlein).

61. What are structured sexual exercises and behavioral modification?

Patients with sexual complaints are always encouraged to make lifestyle modifications. A well-balanced, nutritious diet combined with an active aerobic exercise plan is vital. In fact, vigorous exercise maybe linked to decreased cancer recurrence. Stopping the use of tobacco and illicit drugs, combined with minimizing alcohol consumption, is also encouraged. Take frequent naps, and plan sexual intimacy when you are well rested. Sexual intimacy needs to be a priority for you and your partner. Set limits on other commitments such as employment, social responsibilities, and family obligations. Technology, such as cellular telephones, iPhones, BlackBerries, pagers, and laptop computers, often interferes with private time. If you are preoccupied with these devices, you may be suffering from a **soft addiction**, which can limit intimacy. Limit the use of these devices to a specific time so that they do not hinder sexual intimacy and interpersonal communication.

Similarly, patients may be given specific sexually structured tasks designed to identify and help with specific sexual complaints. Some examples of behavior modification sexual techniques include the following:

- Erotic reading (try reading a racy erotic novel in a quiet, relaxed place!)
- Sensate focusing (concentrate on your physical sensations, notice what feels good when you're intimate with a partner)

- Squeeze-stop technique (alternately tightening and relaxing your pelvic muscles), and stimulation to control ejaculation
- Guided imagery (imagining a particular scenario)
- Relaxation techniques (rhythmic deep and shallow breathing exercises)
- Exploration of sexual fantasies (using props, sexual accessories, or mental imagery)
- **Masturbation**

Many patients are asked to perform sexual exploration, including nongenital touching and self-stimulation exercises, to improve and enhance sexual self-esteem. Patients and their partners are educated through use of open discussions concerning mutual massage, intimate fondling and caressing, or manual, digital, or oral and anal stimulation. Let your imagination be your guide.

Patients and their partners may also be encouraged to engage in alternative sexual positions. Most couples engage in intercourse in the missionary position, which facilitates deep penetration and thrusting. This position, however, can be very painful for the woman who has a shortened vagina in association with vaginal and vulvar atrophy or can place unwelcome pressure on a postoperative surgical site on the chest. Sexual intercourse in alternative positions may include side to side (spooning) or female superior positions, which may help limit deep pelvic thrusting. Other sexual positions encourage direct clitoral stimulation, which greatly facilitates arousal in many women. If movement and mobility are issues (e.g., chronic arthritis, bone and/or joint illness), you can use pillows or down comforters to help create a comfortable sexual environment.

Masturbation
The act of self-pleasuring; also known as self-stimulation.

Tantra

An ancient Indian spiritual tradition and belief system with the premise that sexuality is tied into personal energy and is capable of changing us if we submit to our primal sexual desires while maintaining control and heightening spiritual awareness. Tantra can intensify lovemaking and intensify the sexual dynamic or consciousness between couples.

Tantra is the ancient Indian spiritual tradition and belief system that sexuality is tied to personal energy. It is focused on changing the focus of sexuality from a carnal activity to spiritual enlightenment. Maintaining control and heightening spiritual awareness become the goals of sexual intercourse. When incorporated into love-making, the techniques ultimately intensify the couple's sexual dynamic or consciousness. Sexual enhancement, pleasuring, living consciously, and the various postures of lovemaking are important tenets of Tantra. The union of the yin and yang (the male and female) expands the dimensions of sexuality, and through the control of orgasm, feelings of intimacy and connectedness with your partner are ultimately enhanced.

Pain

When pain is low and fatigue is minimal, sexual expression should be encouraged. Techniques such as warm soaks, physical therapy, and stretching exercises help to loosen tense muscles. Guided imagery, meditation, deep-muscle relaxation, and avoidance of exhaustion are also options. Specifically trained pain management specialists can adjust or reduce opioid regimens, add adjunctive or alternative analgesics, and modify existing dosing schedules, lessening fatigue while maintaining sufficient pain relief.

Sexual Education

Women often are not educated about sexual responsiveness and their genital anatomy. Understanding these will help you know your normal physiological response and how arousal occurs. Examine you genitals with the aid of a hand-held mirror and the assistance of a healthcare professional. Do you know where the clitoral tissue is located? Comprehensive sexuality education may consist of take-home items such as pamphlets, books, videos, and other visual aids. Many widely published resources are available. Many women may opt to search the Internet. The International Society for the Study of Women's Sexual Health, the North American Menopause Society, and the American College of Obstetricians and Gynecologists all maintain wonderful information on their websites about sexual health and education. They also provide medical information about the latest updates on female sexual therapeutics. Please see the resource section for contact information. For the female cancer survivor, the American Cancer Society's booklet *Cancer and Sexuality* is an excellent reference guide that provides helpful suggestions (contact your oncologist or see the Resources).

Magnolia Myrick:

Beware of packaging labeled "natural" and "healthy" because a lot of it is bogus. Educate yourself about reading labels and about nutrition in general. Good information about nutrition is helpful, and it is empowering! It's hopeful.

62. What is sensate focus?

Sensate focus is a term associated with a set of specific sexual exercises for couples or for individuals. It is aimed at increasing personal and interpersonal awareness of our own and our partner's sexual needs. Each participant is encouraged to focus on their own sense experience, rather than to see orgasm as the primary goal of a sexual encounter. A sex therapist will usually guide the timing and technique of the sensate focusing.

In the first stage, the couple is instructed to set aside dedicated time each week to touch each others' bodies, excluding breasts and genitals. They are encouraged to

Sensate focus

A term used to describe a set of sexual exercises for couples or individuals. These exercises are aimed at increasing personal and interpersonal awareness of both our own and our partner's sexual needs.

enjoy and become increasingly aware of the texture and other qualities of their partner's skin. Intercourse and focus on the genitals are disallowed. Participants concentrate on what they find interesting in the skin of the other, not on what they think the other may enjoy.

The second stage of sensate focus increases the areas touched to include breasts. Sensation and gathering information about the partner's body is encouraged, whereas intercourse and touching of the genitals are discouraged. The partners use a "guiding" technique of placing their hand over their partner's hand in order to show what they find pleasurable in terms of pace and pressure. Learning about the partner's body, rather than pleasure, is still the goal. Nonintercourse aspects of sex are explored: touching, tasting, hugging, and kissing. Partners are encouraged to talk to each other, to express emotion, and to encourage one other.

Further stages include the gradual introduction of genitals and then full intercourse; however, intimacy and pleasure, rather than orgasm, remain the primary focus of the couple's interaction. Sensate focus techniques are used for increasing sexual arousal and interest and also as a treatment for sexual dysfunction, especially in sexual difficulties where fear and anxiety are involved.

The aim of sensate focus treatment is to develop an appreciation for an array of sensual possibilities, leading to a reduced concentration on the mechanics of intercourse. Women typically report improved sensation, arousability, and lubrication. Couples often report an improvement in their sex life with less anxiety and greater intimacy.

63. Is it normal to feel uneasy about reading erotic literature?

Many women feel uneasy about reading erotic fantasy literature or viewing sexually explicit films ("porn") to enhance sexual feelings. They may believe that when they read about or view variations in sexual expression or think about sexual activity with a different partner, they are disrespecting or being unfaithful to their "real-life" partner. Fantasy does not necessarily represent one's desire for reality but is simply a means to stimulate parts of the brain where sexual thoughts and behavior originate. Research by world-renowned sexual expert and psychologist Julia Heiman PhD, Director of the Kinsey Institute, suggests that exposure to erotic stories can be a powerful catalyst for a genital engorgement (blood flow, swelling, lubrication) and arousal in both men and women.

Research published by the Sinclair Institute (producers and distributors of erotic films for couples) suggests that female study subjects report increased sexual desire, arousability, and ease of orgasm after viewing erotic scenarios compared with women who viewed sexually neutral films. By considering the use of sexually oriented literature and films as a "self-help" method for sexual vitality, perhaps you can reframe what may have been seen initially as an uncomfortable or shameful activity as a healthy and growth-promoting experience. Discuss exploring sexual **erotica** with your partner and see whether you want to explore this new dimension of sexuality! Look at the Sinclair Institute's website (*www .sinclairinstitute.com*), and order some sexual accessories or videos today—it is a safe, discrete website that can enhance and spice up your sexual life.

Fantasy does not necessarily represent one's desire for reality but is simply a means to stimulate parts of the brain where sexual thoughts and behavior originate.

Erotica

Sexually themed works such as books or sculpture deemed to have literary and artistic merit. Naked men, women, or other body parts are often featured as predominant themes.

64. What pharmacologic interventions can improve sexual function?

Systemic and local estrogen replacement remains key in the management of female sexual dysfunction. Emerging data from the Woman's Health Initiative study describe growing concerns about hormones and potential associated risks of cardiovascular events or breast cancer. Risks and benefit profiles should be discussed with your healthcare and sexual medicine specialist.

Estrogen has many effects on the urogenital system. It promotes **epithelial cell** maturation and proliferation, increases vascularity and blood flow, and stimulates glandular secretions. A decrease of estrogen causes decreased blood supply to the genitals and increased atrophic vaginitis and can lead to painful intercourse and possibly a reactive lowered desire. The use of minimally absorbed local vaginal estrogen (creams, rings, and tablets) for the treatment of vaginal atrophy is widely accepted. Many products are minimally absorbed: Estring (Pfizer) and Vagifem vaginal tablets (NovoNordisk Pharmaceuticals), Premarin Vaginal Cream (Pfizer Pharmaceuticals), and Estrace Cream (Warner Chilcott) and Duramed vaginal Estradiol Cream are other hormonal products that may be used for the vagina and the vulvar tissues. The creams are especially useful for the vulvar and clitoral regions. They can be tapered and used topically in ultra-small amounts. They are widely accepted, cheap, and easy to obtain with a prescription.

Some sexual health providers prefer to prescribe a local 17β-estradiol tablet (Vagifem), which is minimally absorbed into the systemic circulation. Vaginally administered estrogens in small, topically applied doses can be well absorbed. Patients say that the tablets are also easy

Epithelial cell

Any one of several cells arranged in one or more layers that form part of a covering or lining of a body surface.

to use, less messy than cream preparations, and easier to insert than estrogen rings.

Side effects include possible blood clots, increased heart problems, an increase in breast cancer, and increased endometrial cancer if unopposed with a **progestin**. The long-term safety data on minimally absorbed local vaginal estrogen products used in cancer patients remain to be further studied. Talk with your clinician to analyze which one may be right for you.

Progestin

A synthetic form of progesterone often used in birth control pills and hormone therapy.

Women who suffer from atrophy should have an appropriate physical examination. Vaginal atrophy and dryness are relatively easy to diagnose by both a history and physical examination. Women complain of pain, irritation, and discomfort in the vulva and vagina and are fearful of pelvic and digital examinations. After detailed questioning, women often relay additional sexual complaints such as painful intercourse, lowered libido, and increased urinary tract infections. On clinical physical examination, the vagina is dry, pale, frail, and lacks the normal ridges and folds, elasticity, and pliability of a healthy vagina. There is minimal lubrication, and the tissues are easily traumatized with pelvic examination. There can be **petechiae**, or small hemorrhages, on the lining.

Petechiae

Small hemorrhages.

65. What are the common estrogen creams?

Premarin Vaginal Cream (Pfizer) and Estrace Cream (Warner Chicott) contain estrogens that may be used for the vagina and vulvar tissues. They come in a tube and often have plastic applicators. Many women find these products especially soothing to the irritated pelvic area. They can be managed individually using more or less of the product, depending on your situation. The vulvar area, which is sensitive to estrogen levels, can become irritated when hormonal levels are lowered. Women find estrogen creams especially comforting because they can be applied to the external pelvic area as well.

The usual dose is 0.5 g (marked on the applicator) daily for 1 or 2 weeks, and then it is gradually reduced to one half the initial doses for a similar period. A maintenance dose can be used one to three times a week. It may be used after restoration of the vaginal lining has been achieved. You can taper the medication over 3 to 6 months.

Of course, if you experience any side effects, such as vaginal bleeding, while on the cream, speak with your healthcare provider. Newer, lower doses have also been shown to be effective. New recent published data showed good safety with minimal endometrial effects and low systemic absorption with a new lower dose of 0.5 gram two times a week. The FDA has granted approval of Premarin Vaginal Cream for the treatment of moderate to severe vaginal dyspareunia!

An interesting new and exciting use for vaginal estrogen creams is in the field of sexual arousal and orgasms. Recently, the *Journal of Sexual Medicine* published a small case series of women who used estrogen cream applied to the clitoral tissue. These women experienced increased arousal and increased orgasmic intensity. Use cream in the clitoral region if you are suffering from clitoral atrophy or have changes in arousal or orgasm. The use of hormonal creams remains controversial in breast cancer patients and cancer patients are advised to discuss their medical condition with their managing oncological team. Some oncology health care providers have agreed that quality of life concerns and the impact of vaginal dryness can be devastating and have begun to cautiously prescribe local estrogen products to selected patients. Discuss your personal and individual situation with your provider today.

66. What are vaginal estradiol tablets and vaginal rings?

Intravaginal estrogens are applied to the vaginal tissues, and many products are minimally absorbed. Some sexual health providers prefer to prescribe minimally absorbed local 17β-estradiol tablets (NovoNordisk Pharmaceuticals). Vaginally administered estrogens in small, topically applied doses can be well absorbed. Patients say that the tablets are also easy to use, sometimes less messy than cream preparations, and technically easier to insert than estrogen rings. Ultralow doses of vaginal tablets are expected on the market shortly—they allow for vaginal health with minimal systemic effects.

Sometimes vaginal estradiol rings are prescribed for older women who complain of vaginal dryness and painful penetration. Not all vaginal estrogen rings are the same; they vary with respect to absorption into systemic circulation. Many women find them convenient because the rings are placed within the vaginal vault and are not changed for several months. The lower dose vaginal rings release 7.5 micrograms per day of estradiol; this dose produces a steady state of serum (blood) levels of 6–8 pg/mL. This dose can treat local complaints of vaginal dryness but is not sufficient to treat hot flashes or other menopausal symptoms.

According to the North American Menopause Society's recent position statement concerning local vaginal estrogens, rings may change position during bowel movements, douching, and intercourse; however, there is no need to remove the ring during intercourse. In clinical experience, some women and men find rings uncomfortable. No data report on possible allergy to the silasitic plastic ring. Thickening of the endometrium or endometrial hyperplasia usually does not occur until levels surpass 19 pg/mL. The routine addition of a progestational agent is often not used or recommended.

All estrogen products carry a black-box warning and may mention some of the risks or complications. Some of the rare side effects include possible blood clots, increased heart problems, an increase in breast cancer, and increased endometrial cancer if unopposed with a progestin.

67. What is testosterone replacement, and how is it linked with women's sexuality?

Testosterone is also a hormone that remains controversial for women with breast cancer. Many researchers are still unconvinced of any direct link between testosterone and female sexual health. The data are confusing and conflicting. **Female androgen insufficiency syndrome** is characterized by blunted or decreased motivation, persistent fatigue, and a decreased sense of personal well-being that is identified by insufficient plasma estrogen, low circulating bioavailability of testosterone, and low sexual desire (libido). Other potential symptoms include bone loss, decreased muscle strength, and changes in cognition or memory. Bone density may also be affected.

In September 2005, the North American Menopause Society published a comprehensive position statement on

Female androgen insufficiency syndrome

A constellation of symptoms attributed to low testosterone levels in women. Some of the symptoms include fatigue, decreased well-being, a lack of energy or motivation, and decreased or absent sexual interest or desire.

its inclusive review of testosterone use, which included monitoring, safety, and replacement guidelines and doses for postmenopausal women. Currently, no U.S. FDA-approved androgen product is available for women. The use of male products or bioidentical products should be used with caution, as more long-term safety data are warranted. In Europe, the testosterone patch Intrinsa has been recently approved and will be released shortly.

Very high levels of testosterone may have several potentially serious side effects, including increased facial and body hair growth, weight gain, abnormal enlargement of the clitoris, hair loss, changes in lipid profiles, and liver or hematological changes. Women who have taken testosterone supplements have also reported emotional changes. The safety of androgen in the cancer population has not been adequately studied. Testosterone can be converted to estrogen, which may reactivate, promote, or stimulate tumor growth. Intrinsa may be promising for libido issues; however, further randomized controlled trials that examine long-term safety data are warranted.

Some of the testosterones successfully used in women include oral methyl testosterone, transdermal testosterone, topical testosterone propionate cream 2%, testosterone gel, and oral dehydroepiandrosterone. A woman who is taking testosterone off-label in an effort to increase desire or for libido issues should be under the care of a sexual medicine specialist and should have her blood lipids and liver monitored; any side effects should be immediately reported to the clinician.

The authors who conducted a recent study concluded that testosterone replacement in breast cancer patients who are suffering from lowered libido was ineffective. This finding also reiterates that sexual libido is a multivariate problem that involves a complexity of issues, including sexual medicine and sexual psychology.

Women are not ruled by hormones alone. There are women with low or no hormones whose sexual function is excellent and those with hormones that are within the normal range who are sexually dysfunctional.

68. How can phosphodiesterase inhibitors be helpful to women? I thought they were only for men.

Phosphodiesterase inhibitors (medications such as Sildenafil [Viagra], Tadalafil [Cialis], and Vardenafil [Levitra]) are medications that have been used traditionally for the treatment of **erectile dysfunction** in men. Numerous attempts have been made to show an efficacy in women, but most fail to show any significant benefit. The medication is supposed to relax the clitoral and vaginal smooth muscle. Some potential side effects of this class of medications include headache, uterine contractions, dizziness, hypotension, myocardial infarction (heart attack), stroke, and sudden death.

Erectile dysfunction

A persistent or recurrent inability to achieve or maintain an erection sufficient enough to accomplish a desired sexual behavior such as intercourse or coitus.

New and exciting emerging data may support their use in women who suffer from sexual complaints because of selective serotonin reuptake inhibitor (SSRI) use. Recent data suggest that men who use phosphodiesterase inhibitors may actually be helping their spouses achieve sexual satisfaction. In an article titled "Through the Eyes of Women: The Partners' Perspective on Tadalafil," which was published in the *Journal of Urology* in September 2006, Althof and associates attempted to evaluate patient and partner responses to the efficacy and overall satisfaction with use of tadalafil to treat erectile dysfunction. This was a double-blinded, placebo-controlled, 12-week trial of approximately 746 couples who received either placebo or 10 or 20 mg of tadalafil. Female partners of men who were taking the medication reported significantly improved overall sexual satisfaction and corroborated the men's report of erectile improvement and penetration ability. The men were understandably happy, and many reported improved erection, penetration, and overall satisfaction with the sexual experience while taking the medication. Sexual complaints do not exist in an individual vacuum but rather are intricately involve the partner and his or her reaction to treatment.

Some women who have changes in orgasm (it takes too long to achieve an orgasm and the intensity and frequency of orgasm have diminished) may benefit from the use of a phosphodiesterase inhibiting medication. Ask your sexual healthcare provider if this medication may be helpful for you.

69. What is Alprostadil cream?

Alprostadil cream is a prostaglandin E1 cream. It is not FDA approved for the treatment of female sexual dysfunction but has been used in men for the treatment of erectile dysfunction; however, according to preliminary clinical trials, this topical medication (a compounded cream) can be applied to the pelvic genital area in women and may act to relax arterial smooth blood vessels, causing vasodilation and increased sensitivity and sexual arousal. NexMed pharmaceutical company is conducting advanced randomized clinical trials with this cream with the intention of making it widely available in the United States under the brand name Femprox.

A similar product, Alista, is under investigation by Vivus. In a double-blind trial, 400 women with female sexual arousal disorder aged 21 to 65 years were randomized to receive a 10-dose at-home treatment of 500, 700, or 900 μg of Alprostadil cream or a placebo cream. They were instructed to apply the cream to their clitoris and **G-spot**. More than 370 patients completed the study, and many showed significant improvement in sexual arousal. Possible side effects include pain to the genitals (decreased as the cream was washed away), lowered blood pressure, and possible temporary fainting. Alprostadil cream should be topically applied approximately 15 minutes before engaging in intercourse.

G-spot

An area of increased erotic sensitivity on or deep inside the front of the vagina. It is located on the anterior surface of the vaginal vault. Stimulation in some women provides intense sexual pleasure.

70. What is Apomorphine?

Apomorphine has been used sublingually for the treatment of male sexual health concerns. It is sometimes considered an alternative to the phosphodiesterase inhibitors. In a recent *Journal of Sexual Medicine* article, Bechara and associates published an excellent, although small, study titled "A Double Blind Randomized Placebo Control Study Comparing the Objective and Subjective Changes in Female Sexual Response Using Sublingual Apomorphine." This attempted to show the effect of 3 mg of apomorphine in the female response cycle in those women who were diagnosed with orgasmic problems.

This study demonstrates that clitoral blood flow changes in peak velocity were significantly higher in the subjects who took the medication, which theoretically translates into better pelvic blood flow. This phenomenon, when considered in a broader light, would mean changes in arousal and lubrication. These areas were also significantly improved in the Apomorphine group.

The researchers concluded that this medication was beneficial for women with orgasmic problems or complaints. They also propose an anatomic mechanistic model of the function and result of the drug. The side effects and adverse events were low in incidence and were mostly mild and transient. Although this study involved very small numbers, many sexual healthcare professionals are optimistic because the medication is provocative and warrants further rigorous study for the treatment of female sexual complaints. It is not presently available for prescription to female sexual health patients, but studies are ongoing.

71. How can the antidepressant bupropion (Wellbutrin) be helpful to my sexual health?

Bupropion, or Wellbutrin (GlaxoSmithKline), is a non-serotonin reuptake inhibitor antidepressant (medication that has recently been touted as having the least sexual side effects). This medication is a weak blocker of the uptake of the brain chemicals serotonin and norepinephrine and is commonly used in smoking cessation programs. Some patients on this medication report an increase in sexual desire. A typical trial of this medication includes a starting dose of 75 mg that can be increased gradually. Precautions and possible side effects include insomnia, nervousness, and mild to moderate increases in blood pressure, as well as a risk of lowering seizure threshold.

Drs. Seagraves and Clayton published a study titled "Bupropion Sustained Release for the Treatment of Hypoactive Sexual Desire in Premenopausal Women" in the *Journal of Clinical Psychopharmacology*. This landmark study examined women with hypoactive sexual desire disorder in a randomized placebo-controlled trial with increasing doses of bupropion. All measures indicated increased sexual responsiveness and increased sexual arousal, orgasmic completion, and overall sexual satisfaction. The researchers propose a mechanism by which the medication operates and causes positive sexual effects by acting on the **dopamine** and **norepinephrine** pathways.

There are minimal side effects, and most women can tolerate this medication. It has been used extensively by sexual medicine healthcare providers off-label for complaints of low desire and lowered libido.

72. What is Flibanserin?

Flibanserin is a 5-HT1A agonist/5-HT2 antagonist. It is manufactured by a private German company called Boehringer Ingelheim and was initially produced as an antidepressant medication. In the late 1990s, the company developed a molecule called Flibanserin that seemed to relieve stress in rats. Unfortunately, this medication did not do well as an antidepressant. Its half-life is approximately 7 hours and appears to be safe with minimal interactions with other medications.

Flibanserin shows excellent promise for treatment of hypoactive sexual desire disorder in women. Recently in Europe, data showed the results from the premenopausal trials that reiterated excellent tolerance, a low side-effect profile, and increased satisfying sexual events for those women who took the medication. Few withdrew from the study, and many were very satisfied with the

Dopamine

A catecholamine that serves as a neurotransmitter and also as a hormone inhibiting the release of prolactin from the anterior portion of the pituitary gland. It is involved in the neurochemistry of sexual function for both men and women.

Norepinephrine

A catecholamine with dual roles as a hormone and a neurotransmitter.

results. Ongoing trials are underway for the postmenopausal group. The dose was 100 mg taken at nighttime and showed to decrease distress associated with lowered sexual desire. Side effects were transient and mild.

Because this medication is not a hormone, it can hopefully be used for women who have breast cancer. The medication has now completed stage 3 clinical trials, and many sexual healthcare providers assume effectiveness with minimal side effects. This medication acts centrally, and some of the mild side effects includes somnolence fatigue, and sleeplessness. Unfortunately, although the mechanism of how Flibanserin has yet to be clarified, it may modulate several circuits in the brain that may be linked to feelings of enjoyment and pleasure. It may act as a serotonin modulator that restores the balance of this compound. It may restore hormonal balance.

According to the company's spokesperson, one of those brain circuits apparently helps control sexual desire and arousal. The effects of the drugs are not immediate and may take some time to occur. Recently, data from the Rose study, an open label randomized withdrawal study, were presented in Europe and demonstrated increased desire days and increased satisfying sexual events for women on this medication. Boehringer Ingelheim has placed a large investment in this medication. The company launched four major clinical trials, involving 5,000 women in 220 worldwide locations, with the goal of applying approval shortly. Sexual healthcare providers are eagerly awaiting the news of a potential treatment for female hypoactive sexual desire disorder. Flibanserin was featured in an issue of *Business Week* and gained notoriety as the most plausible treatment for hypoactive sexual desire disorder—a first for women's sexual complaints!

There is also a company-sponsored disease registry that will follow many women with Hypoactive Sexual Desire Disorder (HSDD) or troublesome lowered sexual libido over the course of several years. The Southern California Center for Sexual Health and Survivorship Medicine in Newport Beach and the Institute for Pelvic Pain in Philadelphia were chosen as premier vanguard sites. Eligible participants may enroll after the informed consent procedure and are entitled to remuneration. To see whether you are eligible, e-mail info@thesexualhealthcenter.com or call 949-764-9300. In Philadelphia area, the number is 215-863-8100.

73. What is Tibolone?

Tibolone (Livial) is a synthetic hormone-type drug. Livial has been found to increase the risk of recurrence in a randomized trial for patients with breast cancer (particularly if estrogen receptor positive). It is used mainly for **hormone therapy** in postmenopausal women. Tibolone can help relieve symptoms of the menopause transition, including hot flashes, night sweats, mood changes, vaginal dryness, and vaginal irritation. It can also help to prevent bone health issues such as osteoporosis.

Hormone therapy

The use of medications to modify or replace those whose production is decreased or absent in the menopause period.

Many studies over the last 5 years show that Tibolone, a new female hormone, shares many effects with male hormones and may prevent bone problems and lack of sexual desire. Tibolone's cardiovascular effects are much less clear. On the positive side, the drug reduces total cholesterol and harmful triglycerides and slightly lowers low-density lipoproteins (bad cholesterol), but it also lowers high-density lipoproteins (good cholesterol). Many experts are concerned about this mixed picture toward cardiovascular health.

Tibolone (Livial) is available in much of continental Europe and the United Kingdom, but it is not yet available in the United States. The drug may improve desire, but researchers are uncertain of its effect on other parameters of female sexual function. This medication may not be a viable option for women who have breast cancer.

74. What is Bremelanotide?

PT-141 (Bremelanotide) is a melanocortin receptor agonist that was under study and development for the treatment of both male and female sexual complaints. Originally, this medication was developed and tested as a sunless tanning agent but was not effective; however, some subjects reported increased sexual arousal and spontaneous erections. Some serious concerns regarding the benefit and risk ratio of Bremelanotide caused delay in the stage 3 clinical trial regarding some severe changes in blood pressure. The melanocortins are thought to play an important role in female sexual health and functioning. The medication, which was under study and in advanced clinical trials, is a centrally acting drug that can affect the brain. It is a colorless, odorless chemical that is placed within a nasal inhaler and has been used by many women with sexual complaints. Some women who have taken this medication have reported increased warmth or throbbing in the genitals as well as an increased desire to engage in intercourse. A phase 2A pilot clinical study looked at this medication in premenopausal women diagnosed with female sexual dysfunction, and it has not shown encouraging results.

On May 13, 2008, Palatin Technologies, the maker of Bremelanotide, announced that it had discontinued further development of Bremelanotide for the treatment of both male and female sexual dysfunction; however, the company is researching a new compound, PL-6983, that causes significantly lower increases in blood pressure than those seen with Bremelanotide in animal models. There is hope in the future; we should await further studies and publications. In preliminary studies it has shown to increase sexual activity.

75. What nonhormonal and nonmedication regimes can I use for sexual function?

Sometimes women may opt to use other types of treatment (vaginal moisturizers and lubricants) to help their sexual function.

The liberal use of local nonmedicated, nonhormonal vaginal moisturizers (Replens or vitamin E suppositories) can provide relief for the symptoms of vaginal atrophy. These agents are recommended for use two or three times weekly. Women should wear a minipad when using vitamin E suppositories because they may stain undergarments. Feminease and Me Again are made from non-irritating ingredients.

The use of water-based vaginal lubricants with intercourse is also encouraged when vaginal dryness and atrophy are diagnosed; however, vaginal lubricants that contain microbicides, perfumes, coloration, or flavors may irritate the sensitive atrophic vaginal **mucosa**. Lubricate all surfaces as part of foreplay, and be sure to keep lubricant handy in case more is needed. Lubricants may be water or silicone based. Use a lot of lubricant when attempting intercourse if you have vaginal atrophy or dryness.

Mucosa

A surface layer of cells or epithelium that is lubricated by the secretions of mucosal glands.

Some brands of water-based lubricants include Astroglide, Slippery Stuff, GV Slip Inside, Hydra-smooth, Sensua Organic, Probe, and KY Jelly. Silicone-based lubricants include Wet Platinum and Eros Women. Good Clean Love and Almost Naked are organic, safe, and effective. By using these natural lubricants, women avoid vaginal irritation. Read labels, and avoid brands that contain glycerin or parabens (*www.goodcleanlove.com*).

Some other products include: Viacreme® is a topical, water-based lotion with menthol and L-arginine (for more information: *www.viacremedelight.com*) that is advertised as a product to enhance sexual responsiveness in the genital area. It is also thought to increase genital warming and clitoral sensitivity. To date, no human studies have been conducted to prove the efficacy of this product and many patients complain of severe genital burning and irritation after application.

Another arousal product, available from Johnson and Johnson, is K-Y Brand INTENSE. According to their website (*www.k-y.com/intense*), this patent-pending gel formula was shown in a clinical study to enhance female arousal and satisfaction. In consumer studies, 75% of women reported heightened arousal, sexual pleasure, and sensitivity. Massaging K-Y INTENSE directly onto the clitoris, as directed, stimulates sensitivity and creates a gentle warming sensation, increasing female pleasure during intimacy. Have you (or your partner) gently massage a drop (two to four pumps) of the product onto your clitoris.

Dream Cream is a nonprescription vaginal cream that is odorless and colorless and combines with your own lubrication to help stimulate female genital arousal and blood flow. Its primary ingredient is L-arginine. To enhance sexual intimacy and orgasm, rub it into the clitoral region approximately 10 minutes before sexual intimacy. It does not contain any hormones, nor does it contain menthol, which can be irritating to some women. The cream is not FDA approved, nor have there been any rigorous scientific studies to prove its efficacy.

Other less popular agents include Passion Drops, Lioness, Emerita, Natural Curves, and OMY.

76. What are some common sexual devices or accessories?

A woman can purchase many sexual accessories to help stimulate the genitals. Some enhance pleasure, whereas others are part of a complex sexual medicine treatment plan. Let your imagination be your guide, and explore your sexual fantasies with your partner.

Women who have undergone pelvic surgery; breast cancer patients who have sexual pain syndromes, vaginismus, or other concerns about penetration; or those who suffer from vaginal shortening or vaginal narrowing or who have scar tissue that interferes with or prevents penetration and causes vaginal pain often have pelvic discomfort. **Vaginal dilators** may be prescribed and are graded-size vaginal inserts usually made of plastic, glass, or silicone and are often used to facilitate lengthening and widening of the vagina. They may also be used to help stretch vaginal scar tissue that may have contributed to pain and discomfort during vaginal intercourse. Dilators can be used on a regular basis and with water- or hormone-based lubricants. Suggested schedules range from once daily for 10 to 15 minutes to at least three times weekly. Several studies report that ongoing supportive behavioral

Vaginal dilators

Medical applications that can be placed within the vagina to help restore the vaginal tissues so that they are more adaptable.

therapy is instrumental for continued compliance. A formalized dilator program is often used for those who have sexual pain syndromes. Ask your provider if you are a candidate.

How do you use a vaginal dilator? Using the vaginal dilator can help expand the vagina and help stretch radiation changes of tissue fibrosis (such as hardening of the vaginal wall tissue) that may have been caused by cancer therapy. Prepare yourself and your environment for dilator therapy. Make certain that you will have privacy by either locking your door or working with your dilator when you will not be interrupted. Many clinicians advise women to use their dilators in the morning hours just before starting the day for several reasons. At the end of a long busy day with work, family, and social obligations, dilator therapy may seem too consuming. Too often, fatigue and rest supersede sexual rehabilitation. Dilator therapy is also great in the morning because you can jump in the shower if the lubricant was messy and/or has resulted in any vaginal leakage. The dilator should be inserted into the vagina with a generous amount of lubricant.

You should lie on your back, bend your knees, and spread your knees apart. With gentle pressure, the vaginal dilator should be inserted into the vagina as deeply as possible while still maintaining some comfort. You should leave the dilator in place for 10 to 15 minutes while remaining on your back. It is often helpful to be distracted by other activities (e.g., reading a book or watching television) while the dilator is in place. After removing the dilator, it is important to wash it with soap and warm water, dry it with a clean towel, and store it in a safe, secure place (adapted from the Memorial Sloan-Kettering Cancer Center's patient education materials).

77. What are some common sexual devices that I can use?

The Eros Clitoral Therapy Device (Nugyn) has been prescribed for patients who have had cervical and other pelvic cancers (e.g., rectal and vaginal cancers). It is a battery operated device and has a small vacuum suction that attaches around the clitoral area. It is designed to facilitate engorgement or vasocongestion in the clitoral tissue. Preliminary data showed that this device may be helpful in combating arousal difficulties after cervical cancer therapy. The device may also be helpful for women with arousal or orgasmic disorders or orgasmic problems. It is possible that this device can be helpful in women who complain of changes in orgasmic intensity and latency. It has not been studied in breast cancer patients. It is costly and is available only by prescription. Medical insurance plans vary as to whether they will cover the expense.

What about commercially available vibrators or self-stimulators? Vibrators come in a variety of shapes, sizes, and colors. These sexual devices can be helpful for women who may need extra vibratory stimulation in the sensitive erotic areas of both the vagina and clitoris. Vibrators have proven useful during self-stimulatory behavior and can also be used during sexual foreplay. They are available at local pharmacies, on the Internet, and at local sexual paraphernalia shops. Self-stimulators can be used with water-based lubricants. It is important to keep them clean; wash them with soap and warm water using a sponge or cloth and rinse well. Store them in a clean, dry and private place.

Vibrators can be used alone as part of self-erotic exploration and sexual play or as part of your sexual repertoire with your partner. Generally, sexual massagers can be used both internally and externally to enhance stimulation, arousal, and pleasure. You can stimulate the labia, vaginal tissue, and clitoral tissue and even enhance testicular or penile stimulation for your partner. If you share your sexual toys, then it is doubly important to cleanse them in between each person's use.

One website, *www.drugstore.com*, offers home delivery of sexual accessories in a discrete manner, and you will not receive any unwanted e-mails or mailings.

The Lelo line of self-stimulators includes high-end European sexual stimulator products named Gigi and Liv. They are elegant and highly functional, have multiple speeds, and are very quiet.

The Ohmibod vibrators (*www.ohmibod.com*) combine music and self-stimulation and are helpful for the woman who is suffering from dyspareunia or painful intercourse. The vibrator plugs into your iPod, and as you listen to soothing relaxing music, you can have your mind distracted and allow your body to focus on self-pleasuring without the distraction or fear of pain. Music therapy can be combined to treat vaginismus and other sexual pain syndromes

One new self-stimulator, the Adonis, created by sexual expert Dr. Laura Berman, has gained popularity because it actively stimulates both the clitoral region and the vaginal G-spot. The electronic stimulation device called Slight Touch is a battery-operated, over-the-counter device that applies electrodes to the top of the foot above the ankles and above the buttocks to stimulate nerve pathways to the genital areas. The Vivelle device is a battery-operated external clitoral stimulation device that is worn on the fingers and may help orgasm. It is used with a special lubricant and is available over the counter. Some other very popular female sexual devices include The Rabbit and The Pocket Rocket. Both have been reported to enhance sexual stimulation and orgasmic intensity.

Another excellent self-stimulator is the petit pink, from the Sinclair Institute. It is a pink soft-touch special massager that is compact and powerful; it delivers three vibration speeds. It fits comfortably within the palm of your hand and is also discreet for travel. An added benefit is that a portion of the proceeds from the sale of this product go to support the fight against breast cancer. The Sinclair Institute also has a variety of educational videos and DVDs that come in both explicit and nonexplicit versions. Some helpful titles include *Great Sex for a Lifetime*, *Sexual Imagination*, *8 Ways to Spice It Up*, and the *Better Sex Series*. For more information on how to order these products, visit their website at *www.sinclairinstitute.com*.

Magnolia Myrick:

I think of myself as a fairly modern gal, but I somehow missed the memo on vibrators until I was in my 40s. Yo. Maybe I thought I didn't need one or was too big a prude to use one, let alone buy one—I don't know. But good heavens, why wouldn't any woman want to have an entire collection? They're great! My partner and I use one during sex; he loves it and I love it. What's not to love? There is a vibrator called the "Pocket Rocket," which is a good basic—small, battery-operated, nothing fancy. The Internet is rife with sources. You take it from there, sister.

78. Can alternative and complementary medicine improve my sex life?

Some women have tried many nonconventional sexual enhancers and therapies in order to facilitate treatment for sexual function complaints and arousal disorders. Many products claim to improve sexual function, and some alternative therapies may contain dangerous ingredients and serious side effects and can interfere with prescription medications. Most of these products have not been adequately studied for safety with respect to breast cancer patients. Discuss all supplements with your oncological healthcare team before taking any herbs or supplements.

Discuss all supplements with your oncological healthcare team before taking any herbs or supplements.

Some studies show that a low level (50 mg/day) of dehydroepiandroster (DHEA) can improve the frequency of sexual thoughts, sexual interest, sexual satisfaction, and libido. It can also act like a hormone. This can increase androgens, decrease **high-density lipoproteins (HDL)**, and decrease sex hormone binding globulin, and high levels of DHEA are correlated with increased risk of cardiovascular disease. These products are not monitored by the FDA, and label claims may not accurately reflect the actual DHEA content in the product. The safety of this product has not been adequately studied in breast cancer patients; thus, be sure to discuss this product with their healthcare provider before trying it.

High-density lipoproteins (HDL)

A complex of lipids and proteins in approximately equal amounts that functions as a transporter of cholesterol within the bloodstream.

Avlimil is an herbal 756 mg/day supplemental tablet consisting of sage leaf, red raspberry leaf, capsicum pepper, licorice root, bayberry fruit, damiana leaf, valeriana root, ginger root, black cohosh root, isoflavones, kudzu root extract, and red clover extract (see *www.avlimil.com*). Sage, kudzu, red clover licorice, and black cohosh are known to have estrogenic effects and were used in the past for the treatment of menopausal hot flashes and other symptoms.

Aphrodisiac

A substance believed to improve or enhance sexual function or pleasure. Some think it may stimulate feelings of love, intimacy, or desire.

Damiana leaf has been said to act as an **aphrodisiac**, but no scientific data support this claim. The product package insert states that it is a nonsynthetic, nonhormonal supplement that does not contain estrogen, progesterone, testosterone, or steroid hormones; however, the fine print of the labeling states that "if estrogen levels are low, isoflavones are reported to act as 'weak estrogens.'" Avlimil is presumed to increase sexual satisfaction by increasing genital pelvic blood flow and promoting relaxation. A small, unpublished trial of fewer than 50 women claims a positive effect on female sexual response. Side effects can include headaches, insomnia, anxiety, and stomach upset.

Medulla oblongata

An area of the brain.

Xzite is a daily dietary supplement that claims to stimulate the brain centrally at the level of the **medulla oblongata**, facilitating elevated mood and increased blood flow to the female genital pelvis. Its ingredients include ligusticum, acathopanax, and chrysanthemum. One unpublished study showed improvement in vaginal lubrication, clitoral sensation, orgasmic satisfaction, and sexual desire.

Arginmax (*www.arginmax.com*) is a daily supplement that claims to enhance a woman's sexual response by promoting genital pelvic blood flow and relaxation. It is a blend of L-arginine, Korean ginseng, ginkgo biloba, damiana, calcium, iron, and 14 vitamins. The product claims to increase smooth muscular relaxation, promote vascular dilation, and enhance clitoral engorgement and vaginal lubrication. One very small published study showed an improvement in sexual desire, clitoral sensation, and frequency of orgasms, satisfaction, and increased frequency of sexual intercourse. This product is not adequately studied for safety in the breast cancer population.

Libidol is another daily supplement that consists of sage leaf, red raspberry leaf, kudzu root extract, red clover extract, capsicum pepper, licorice root, bayberry fruit, damiana leaf, valerian root, ginger root, black cohosh root, L-arginine, horny goat weed, and wild oats. Its claims of improving female sexual dysfunction have not been scientifically proven.

Other neutriceuticals and botanicals include avena sativa, catuaba, St. Johns wort, red sage, angus castus, bethroot, calendula, black cohosh, burdock, dong quai, deer antler, eurycoma longifolic, chaste berry, comfrey, fenugreek, evening primrose oil, fennel, licorice root, red clover, raspberry leaf, ginger, horny goat weed, rhino horn, royal jelly, saw palmetto, wild yam zinc, koala nut, maca, and ginseng.

Another interesting supplement is called Hot Plants. It is a compilation of a variety of herbs that have been known in ancient civilizations to improve sexuality and sexual wellness in women. It too has not been studied for effectiveness or safety in women who have had breast cancer.

79. Do diet or nutrition improve sexual function?

Although patients try many different foods, such as chocolate, ginseng, oysters, and popular sex-enhancing diets, to facilitate improved sexual function, none has been shown in randomized clinical trials to be beneficial for correcting female sexual complaints. Some of the more popular diets include the following:

- The Orgasmic Diet includes avoidance of antidepressants, coffee, tea, caffeine, soft drinks, cigarettes, herbal stimulants, ginkgo, and ginseng. It also adds a multivitamin with vitamin E (400 mg), vitamin C,

6-g fish oil (omega-3), calcium (100 mg), magnesium (400 mg), zinc (15 mg), and slow-release iron. Women are encouraged to maintain a low-carbohydrate diet, perform **Kegel pelvic exercises**, and consume one ounce of dark chocolate daily.

- The Testosterone Diet consists of nuts, olive oil, canola oil, peanut butter, turnips, broccoli, cabbage, mustard greens, Brussels sprouts, radishes, collard greens, watercress, and bok choy. Avoid all alcohol, and maintain good sleep patterns and regular aerobic exercise.

- The Gladiator Diet includes weight-lifting exercise and a diet void of alcohol, sweets, and processed foods while ingesting a balanced diet consisting of 33% each of calories from carbohydrates, fats, and proteins.

Aphrodisiacs have been heralded since ancient times as a way to enhance sexual performance and improve desire; however, scientific and medical data are lacking. Some of the more commonly accepted food aphrodisiacs include oysters, lobster, mussels, horseradish, lettuce, carrots, celery, caffeine, mustard seeds, radishes, wine, champagne, truffles, and spices (nutmeg, cayenne pepper, cinnamon, coriander, basil, clover, cardamom, and honey).

Chocolate is often associated with romance, apology, and seductive gifts. It does contain biogenic amines, tyramine, phenylethamine (the so-called love drug), methylxanthines, and cannabinoid-like fatty acids. Chocolate is also thought to enhance or promote sensuality and improve sexual function or virility. Unfortunately, a recent study published in the *Journal of Sexual Medicine* failed to find an association between the consumption of chocolate and sexual function.

Kegel pelvic exercise

Exercise designed to increase muscle strength and elasticity in the pelvis. It may be recommended in the treatment of urinary incontinence.

Although not linked to improved sexual function, the new and innovative supplement Juice Plus Orchard Blend and Juice Plus Garden Blend have been gaining popularity in the breast cancer population. They have been researched extensively, and many researchers claim that they have excellent medical and antioxidant properties. These supplements are advocated for many medical reasons, including reducing inflammation, fighting obesity, improving cholesterol, fighting cancers, and preventing breast cancer or its reoccurrence. For further information, contact your oncological healthcare provider.

80. What is Zestra Essential Arousal Oil?

Zestra® Essential Arousal Oils™ is a topically-applied, patented blend of botanical oils and extracts that is clinically proven to improve desire, arousal, and satisfaction for 70% of women. The active ingredients are natural and include Zestra's unique formulation of PA-free borage seed oil, evening primrose oil, angelica Extract, coleus forskholii extract as well as theobromine, and the antioxidants Vitamin C and Vitamin E. Zestra's botanical ingredients work together to safely and effectively enhance female sexual pleasure, sensation, sensitivity, and satisfaction.

The author's clinical experience finds that Zestra helps many women achieve sexual wellness, increased arousal, and overall sexual and sensual satisfaction. The use of Zestra results in increased clitoral and vaginal warmth, heightened arousal, and increased sexual pleasure in selected women.

Zestra's safety and effectiveness has been demonstrated in two clinical studies, both published in the peer-reviewed

Journal of Sex and Marital Therapy in 2003 and 2010. The first study, a small clinical trial involved 20 women—10 of the women in the study had sexual concerns and difficulties and 10 did not. Most of the women (with or without sexual concerns or difficulties) experienced benefits from Zetsra. The 2nd larger study with 256 women supported the earlier findings. The larger study included women in a range of ages and life stages, reflecting a variety of sexual difficulties and medical histories, including women on anti-depressants and in various stages of menopause. Zestra worked equally well for women regardless of their medical history, medication usage or menopausal status. The author has had clinical success using Zestra with cancer patients and those in treatment. The ongoing use seems to have a positive affect on sensation.

Zestra can increase vaginal and clitoral warmth for up to 30 to 45 minutes after a single application, facilitating sexual arousal and ultimately leading to increased pleasure. Mild genital burning has been reported. Borage and evening primrose oils can be metabolized in the skin to increase blood flow and nerve conduction. Semprea Laboratory which owns and distributes the product have coined the term the Zestra Rush! The authors have submitted a case abstract of breast cancer survivors who have had success with this product to an international sexual medicine society, more exciting news about this product is forthcoming! For more information go to *www.zestra.com.*

81. Can acupuncture increase libido?

Acupuncture and herbal Chinese medicine incorporate more than 2,000 years of experience in treating sexual dysfunction. Multiple studies have concluded that when acupuncture needles are placed in specific key locations of the body, many processes are activated, including hormone release, nervous system regulation, and increased vascular blood flow. Acupuncture also has a profound calming effect on mental and emotional states, thus enhancing feelings of well-being and sexual desire.

Acupuncture has been used for several hundred years to treat a variety of medical concerns, including pelvic pain, headaches, menopausal hot flashes, and anxiety. The authors have developed an acupuncture and herbal medicine program that specifically addresses the concerns of women who are suffering from lowered libido. It has been very helpful for women with breast cancer who have hot flashes and lowered libido. Our comprehensive approach couples Eastern and Western medical practices. The acupuncturist typically takes a comprehensive history. An individualized management plan is created, and ongoing care often yields excellent results. Traditional Chinese medicine specialists feel that sex drive and desire are from **Yuan Chi**. According to the book *Chi and Libido* by Tom Tam, Yuan Chi is defined as the genuine chi and can be thought of as the life essence provided at conception by both parents. Yuan Chi is housed in the kidney, and its primary function is to promote normative bodily growth and development, as well as to maintain the health and vigor of all bodily functions. With time, Yuan Chi can be diminished by a variety of different issues such as poor diet, excessive lifestyle, stress, and diseases such as cancer and their subsequent treatments.

Yuan Chi

The genuine chi and can be thought of as the life essence provided at conception by both parents.

When considering the complex issue of sexual function in women, treatment must be tailored to the patterns of imbalance that are revealed through tongue and pulse diagnosis, as well as detailed history concerning diet, lifestyle, and medical and emotional health.

133

Acupuncturists are specialized healthcare professionals who are required to complete 4 years of academic and clinical training before becoming eligible to take the rigorous state and licensing examinations.

Acupuncturists are specialized healthcare professionals who are required to complete 4 years of academic and clinical training before becoming eligible to take the rigorous state and licensing examinations. Strict standards are required to maintain their licenses. Needles, when used, are under strict healthcare regulations for maintaining sterile environments.

82. Can exercise improve sexual function?

Besides the obvious health reasons, numerous recent studies have shown that regular exercise can remarkably improve sexuality. Exercise has also been linked to decreased breast cancer rates. Exercise may enhance sexual performance and decrease sexual dysfunction from physical, physiologic, and psychological perspectives. A frequent and intense exercise program that focuses on cardiovascular and muscular endurance, muscular strength, and flexibility can allow for longer lasting and more comfortable sex.

One sexual encounter actually burns 50–200 calories, which is comparable to one to three small chocolate chip cookies. Physical exercise improves physiologic sexual response and functioning by increasing circulation, which includes blood flow to the genital region. A recent study conducted by Cindy Meston at the University of Texas at Austin shows that when women have exercised vigorously for 20 minutes they are more quickly aroused than without exercise. Exercise has also been shown to reduce stress, improve self-esteem, and increase a personal sense of confidence. These positive psychological effects cause you to feel good about your personal, physical, and sexual attractiveness and ability.

Exercise is an important aspect for breast cancer survivorship because many studies have shown that improved exercise plans and vigorous exercise can be associated with decreased disease recurrence. Consult an exercise specialist and begin a new exercise plan today! You, your heart, and your love life will be happy you did!

Magnolia Myrick:

I decided that even if I went to the gym and laid down on the treadmill, I was getting my behind in there. People think cancer patients always lose weight. Wrong! If you're having chemo and all you feel like eating is macaroni and cheese, guess what? I upped my training sessions to three days a week—a luxury not all budgets or schedules allow, I realize, but that is no excuse for doing nothing. A structured program, something or someone that compels you to show up is best, no doubt, but anything is better than nothing. The hardest thing about exercising is beginning. Put on those sneakers and walk out the door. Even if you just go around the block, good! Bet you'll go further, though. I came to see exercise as essential not just to my overall recovery and fitness, but to my confidence, energy, and sense of well-being. All this stuff is scientifically documented, of course, but I'm telling you, it's the best thing you can do for yourself. It makes everything better. Go at your own pace, and do what you can. You will amaze yourself. And you know what? During treatment, I definitely had some days that were better than others, but I never did lie down on that treadmill.

83. What is mindfulness training?

Many of us travel on preprogrammed, unthinking autopilot—going to work, going through the motions without really paying attention to our surroundings or reactions. Often we are actually deep into a phase of life often called "mindlessness." We go home, check e-mail, cook dinner, and attend to the children. Undoubtedly, we shoot off e-mail messages containing spelling errors or reply harshly without thought or consideration. We cut our fingers chopping lettuce or miss the joyful smile of the coy, crafty toddler getting into mischief. We are on overload. The habit of inattention, going through the motions, or having your brain race with thoughts leads us to never be present in our daily lives. We often ignore or dismiss important information and messages from our relationships, our friends, our own health, and even our own life. We can zone out, tune out, and shut out the world almost automatically when stress invades our lives.

Practicing the art of mindfulness is the key to being in the present moment—using all of your focused senses in a challenged dynamic thought process. Sight, smell, touch, taste, and hearing all work in unison to create a whole image and picture of the process. Stop and smell the roses, but appreciate the hue of redness, the texture of the leaves, the imperfections of the petals, and the sparkling fragrance of the unique flower.

Dr. Lori Brotto, noted sexual health researcher, and some of her Vancouver colleagues have published extensively on the notion of mindfulness and its use in the treatment of female sexual dysfunction disorders. The concept of focusing on bodily functions and performance can help women a great deal in understanding their bodies' normal function. Intense focusing on self can also help to solidify and enhance sexual constructs and thoughts. Brotto and her colleagues have shown this technique of mindfulness training to be effective in patients with malignancies, sexual complaints, a variety of other medical conditions, and chronic pain syndromes.

Try some relaxation techniques such as deep breathing and resting comfortably in quietness. Pay attention without letting your mind wander or trying to change any thought. Be aware. Stop and smell and touch and feel and appreciate the rose petals in their universe and specific environmental context. Stay in the present, and if you wander, let yourself drift back to your original thought. Focus on your deep breathing, each breath as it enters and exits your lungs, before an activity, and think about the experience. You can expect your mind to wander or deviate from the concentration course with intrusive or conflicting thoughts, but slowly, thoughtfully, and gently bring it back to the concentrated ideal or experience. Try to anchor your awareness in the present moment. Stay focused, and try not to let your mind wander on to the future or the "what-ifs" that life may bring. Begin by trying to narrow your focus of thought and to appreciate your individual thoughts and ideals. Your mind will become clearer and senses more heightened. You will be in the moment during sexual intimacy and feel a deeper sense of connection both to your inner sexual self and your partner's sensuality. Do not expect to achieve a state of mindfulness overnight—it is a process of practice and dedication. The more you focus your mind and channel your energies, the easier it will become for future endeavors. Yoga, meditation, and even acupuncture may be helpful in the treatment of sexual complaints. New data are emerging about these stress and relaxation techniques, and many find help by incorporating them into their treatment plans.

PART FIVE

Reestablishing and Strengthening Your Sexual Relationship

Is it normal for couples to put less emphasis on their sexual relationship while undergoing surgery, chemotherapy and/or radiation?

What if I am having trouble reestablishing a sexual relationship with my partner after treatment is over?

How do I communicate to my partner what has changed in my body?

More . . .

84. Is it normal for couples to put less emphasis on their sexual relationship while undergoing surgery, chemotherapy, and/or radiation?

Research suggests that during treatment for breast cancer it is very common for couples to de-emphasize their sexual relationship and prioritize "making it through the fatigue, nausea, and surgical recuperation." Women and their partners may have fearful thoughts of loss and even death during this time, and mental health challenges such as depression, anxiety, and difficulty coping can impact simple activities of daily living.

Weeks, months, and sometimes years after the acute phase of the cancer experience has passed (when "life is getting back to normal"), the subject of return to sexual intimacy may arise. You may not feel sexual but may want to cuddle or be held. You may only want to kiss, but other forms of sexual activity are not in your mind. Discuss your concerns with your lover or partner.

After a prolonged period of supportive but relatively platonic interaction, either or both members of the couple may find it very awkward to talk about and/or initiate sexual activity.

85. What if I am having trouble re-establishing a sexual relationship with my partner after treatment is over?

After a prolonged period of supportive but relatively platonic interaction, either or both members of the couple may find it very awkward to talk about and/or initiate sexual activity. The longer the couple struggles with this awkwardness, the longer it can be before intimacy returns. Many couples find it difficult to restart sexual activity and thus consult with their healthcare provider or a sexual specialist for assistance. The boundaries of what will feel good and what may be uncomfortable can no longer be assumed.

A sexual specialist can help a woman living with breast cancer and her sexual partner identify and address aspects of their sexual life (many that they have never had to overtly address during their entire relationship) and make suggestions about having a sexual dialogue, as well as about which lubricants, moisturizers, prescription medications, foreplay techniques, and sexual positions are best. This is often a wonderful time that promotes a sexual growth experience.

86. What "self-help" techniques allow women get their desire back?

It is normal for many women to "never feel in the mood spontaneously." Most women who are dealing with a health issue report that they need to "psyche themselves up" to be physically intimate. There are many ways of augmenting desire.

Some specific strategies include reading erotic stories, watching sexy films, using vibrators or stimulators to self-pleasure, and fantasizing about erotically charged times in the past. When women use these techniques, they are helping to enhance something known as **reactive desire**, which is the type of motivation for sex that happens when a woman says "yes" to a sexual invitation from a partner (even if she initially feels no initial interest or motivation for physical contact). After the sexual activity begins, however, she may begin to feel increasingly aroused and invested in the intimate activity. She may seek sexual closeness for a variety of reasons, not only

Reactive desire

Desire that is triggered from an external stimuli rather than occuring spontaneously.

sexual hunger or innate desire but often because of the urge to be close with her partner.

Many women report that "it's only after things get going for a while that I start to think sexual thoughts. I start thinking that physical closeness is a good idea…I begin to enjoy the sensations and want them to continue."

Reactive desire is facilitated most when a woman stays focused in the moment during intimacy and doesn't let her mind wander to household, childrearing, or work issues. The renowned sex therapist team of Dr. Barry McCarthy and his wife, Emily McCarthy, have suggested the following guidelines for revitalizing sexual desire:

- The keys to sexual desire are positive anticipation and feeling that you deserve sexual pleasure.
- Each person is responsible for his or her desire with the couple functioning as an intimate team to nurture and enhance desire. Revitalizing sexual desire is a couple function; guilt and blame subvert the change process.
- Inhibited desire is the most common sexual dysfunction, affecting one in three couples. Desire problems drain intimacy and good feelings from the relationship.
- The initial romantic love/passionate sex pattern of desire lasts less than 2 years and often less than 6 months. Desire is facilitated by an intimate, interactive sexual relationship.
- The essence of sexuality is giving and receiving pleasure-oriented touching. The prescription to revitalize and maintain sexual desire is intimacy, pleasuring, and eroticism.

- Touching should occur both inside and outside the bedroom. Touching does not always have to lead to intercourse.

- Couples who maintain a healthy sexual relationship use touching in many ways. One is affectionate touch (holding hands, kissing, hugging). Another is nongenital, sensual touch, which can be clothed, semiclothed, or nude (body massage, cuddling on the couch, showering together, touching going to sleep or on awakening). Another is playful touching, which intermixes genital and nongenital touching—this can be in bed, dancing, or on the couch clothed or unclothed. Another is erotic touching (manual, oral, or rubbing) to high arousal and orgasm for one or both partners. The last form integrates pleasurable and erotic touch, which flows into intercourse.

- Both partners should value affectionate, sensual, playful, erotic, and intercourse experiences.

- Both partners should be comfortable initiating touching and intercourse. Both should feel free to say no and suggest an alternative way to connect and share pleasure.

87. How do I know when it's time to consult a professional?

Sometimes couples feel ill-prepared to address an interpersonal problem with which they have had no past experience and feel that it is too big to tackle on their own. Redefining what constitutes satisfying sex after cancer can be one such task. If this is the case, you are not alone; many couples benefit from a short course of sex therapy. Sexual health and vitality is a right for anyone regardless of disease or status of chronic medical condition.

Seek a professional if you and your partner have tried resuming your previous ways of being sexual with one another (verbally and nonverbally) and something is not working or not as you had assumed it would. Perhaps your partner is fearful of hurting you and is looking for clues (rather than asking) about what feels good and what doesn't. Perhaps you are both struggling with the change in appearance of the body or sensitivity of your breasts or genitals. All of these are very common themes among couples who may need assistance from a sexual healthcare provider.

88. What is sex therapy?

A certified sex therapist, sometimes referred to as a behavioral sexologist, is an individual with advanced training in the psychosexual and behavioral management of sexual concerns that may stem from a myriad of circumstances, including cancer treatment and survival. A sex therapist can provide sexuality education, individual and couples counseling and support, instruction, and direction in specific techniques for symptom management. A treatment course in sex therapy is usually brief and goal directed as well as highly effective.

Certified sexual therapists often work in close collaboration with the medical healthcare team and will (with your consent) discuss your case with the other specialists. Sex therapists are particularly valuable if you have concerns related to body image and sexual self-esteem, couples communication, a lack of sexual desire, or sexual pain.

89. How do I communicate to my partner about what has changed in my body?

Begin by starting the dialogue with comments such as, "I am really looking forward to being intimate with you again, but I am a little nervous about the differences in my body."

A woman can actually anticipate and address her partner's questions and concerns. Being honest about sexual fears is the first step in conquering them. Research confirms that partners want to discuss sexuality and intimate concerns but may feel that they don't know the right words or appropriate timing. People want to share their concerns but are not sure when to do so. They will likely have no problem modifying their styles to maximize pleasure and minimize discomfort, but they may not be able to anticipate the specific ways that will be helpful for their spouse. By making specific suggestions, you can communicate your individual needs and move toward sexual wellness. Examples of specific comments include

- "For now, please avoid touching my incision site because it is very sensitive."
- "Don't be afraid to touch my breasts. There is no pain, and I really enjoy that closeness."
- "I need to take some time before we make love to put on some special lubricant because my hormones have changed and I don't get as wet as I used to."
- "I want you inside of me but I can only handle about 5 minutes of intercourse before I start to feel sore. We might have to stop and finish another way. Is that okay?"

Honest communication about sexual changes decreases misunderstandings and helps you and your partner work together.

90. What can I do to make sex more comfortable?

The first choice for breast cancer survivors is to use a combination of vaginal moisturizers and vulvar lubricants. In addition, you may want to take your pain medication about 20 to 30 minutes before anticipated sexual activity. Also, use pillows and support cushions during sexual intercourse. When intimate, find a position where pain and discomfort are minimal.

For many breast cancer survivors, there is an undeniable link between their hormonal status, painful sexual activity, bladder symptoms, and the development of a muscle spasm in the pelvic floor muscles, which are a group of muscles that support the bladder, the genitals, and the bowel. They are under both voluntary (the muscles you can squeeze to hold back urine flow or to do a "Kegel" exercise) and involuntary control (they maintain a certain baseline tone in order to support the organs and bones of the pelvis).

Sometimes, fear of repeated soreness with sex can cause a woman to involuntarily brace her pelvic muscles, as if to "guard" herself from painful penetration. Over time, this tightening can become a sustained guarding response, and the muscles can actually shorten and be unable to stretch enough to accommodate a penis or a vibrator comfortably, leading to more pain. Several strategies can help women with hypertonic pelvic floor muscle spasm (also called vaginismus). Most sexual medicine experts are able to examine a woman and perform measurements to evaluate her pelvic floor muscles. If she demonstrates a sustained guarding of her muscles, she may receive a prescription for an oral or intravaginal suppository form of a muscle relaxant (e.g., diazepam, carisoprodol, and cyclobenzaprine). If this fails to relax her muscles sufficiently, she may be directed to a pelvic floor physical therapist, who is specially trained in exercises to strengthen the core muscles of the body and relax and stretch the pelvic floor muscles. The physical therapist may work externally on the muscles of the abdomen, low back and buttocks, as well as inside the vagina, performing an internal massage technique. Although this may seem unusual, pelvic floor physical therapists are usually women who are fully trained in these techniques and take the utmost care to maintain a professional and private therapy environment. Finally, after either or both of these steps, a woman and/or her partner can be taught to reeducate the vaginal muscle by inserting a series of graduated-sized medical dilators (covered with lubrication) into the vagina for 10 minutes several times per week. This facilitates the muscles stretching and then maintaining the proper tone to accommodate comfortable sexual intercourse.

91. How does novelty affect sex drive and responsiveness?

When it comes to looking for ways to spice up the romantic interest and sexual drive in a relationship, breast cancer survivors are similar to all other women, for whom maintaining motivation for intimacy and connection may be a constant challenge. Most studies of love and marriage show that romantic love and its attendant sexual "pizzazz" decline in all relationships over time.

When it comes to looking for ways to spice up the romantic interest and sexual drive in a relationship, breast cancer survivors are similar to all other women, for whom maintaining motivation for intimacy and connection may be a constant challenge.

The excitement of early romance tends to fade and is replaced by familiarity and predictability. You are aware of your sexual script. You know what happens from the start to orgasm and things progress without surprise or excitement. Sexual play is boring and predictable, as if the sequence of events is set in motion and happens almost spontaneously.

When couples do new and exciting things together, their emotional and sexual bonds with each other may be strengthened. The goal for couples interested in enriching their romantic lives, according to Dr. Helen Fisher, anthropologist and romantic love expert, is to find ways of regularly increasing novelty in the relationship, causing a rise in brain chemicals related to sexual interest, drive, and feelings of romantic love for a partner. It also helps the connectedness or intimate bond between partners.

Dr. Arthur Aron, professor of social psychology, suggests that rather than visiting familiar restaurants, dining with the same friends, ordering the same meals, couples who are interested in "spicing up" their romantic lives should plan special date nights that involve new and different activities that they both enjoy. The novel activities need not be exotic or expensive and can be as simple as trying a new type of cuisine, visiting an art exhibit, or going to a county fair. Dance around naked in the living room. Listen to music, or plan an activity that is new for both of you!

Magnolia Myrick said:

Planning sexual excitement doesn't cost much money—your imagination is the only needed tool. Let your mind wander and explore new and different exciting sensual and sexual aspects of your sexual function. Improve the communication between yourself and your partner!

All this talk about vibrators and sexy books and movies might just send you running. But listen, if whatever you're doing is not working, you need to try something else. If you can get over yourself, and you can, and try any of these spicing-up techniques here, you will love it. So will your partner—trust me. And lighten up, if you haven't already. What all these serious medical people might not tell you is not to take yourself too seriously. It is their job to take you seriously, so they can take some of the pressure off you. It may well be that the less seriously you can approach this whole sex business, the better. When you think about it, sex is nothing if not hilarious. (I mean think about it. Are you thinking about it? Are you laughing now? Good.)

I always thought I had a pretty good sex life, and one of the most frightening things about cancer to me was the prospect of losing my desire and my sex appeal. (Well, that and dying, of course.) Using some of the techniques described throughout this book, I practiced to keep the home fires burning. Yes, my body's changed; the vagina is drier and sometimes gets sore after sex. And no, I don't want to "Do It" as often as I used to. But honestly, now 6 years post-diagnosis, post-menopause, and in my early 50s, I am having the best sex I ever had. Some of it has to do with my own growth and development, I'm sure. A lot of it has to do with my wonderful partner. He encourages me, and us, to be adventurous, to use vibrators, to tell sexy stories, to have fun in the sack, and to laugh. Laughing is about the sexiest thing I know.

92. How can it be possible to change brain chemicals with simple behaviors?

Dr. Fisher's research is based on brain medical science. Her research found that new experiences activate the brain's reward system, flooding it with neuro brain chemicals called dopamine and norepinephrine. The reward system area of the brain is the same area that is flooded with chemicals when a person first "falls in love." The result is several symptoms that may feel very familiar to you as you recall when you first felt romantic feelings for someone. "Can't eat, can't sleep, think about them all the time, yearn to be together 24 hours a day, wanting to be united physically, emotionally, spiritually...." Actually, it is similar to obsessive-compulsive behavior (the same brain chemicals are involved in that diagnosis, too!).

Dr. Aron has tested the novelty theory in a series of experiments with long-term married couples. In his studies, couples completed questionnaires about their relationship before and after a series of assigned tasks. Some couples were assigned a somewhat boring task, such as walking back and forth across a room, whereas others were challenged with novel and physically exertional tasks involving crawling and pushing a ball while their wrists and ankles were immobilized. Results indicated that couples who took part in the more challenging exercise tasks showed greater increases in love and satisfaction survey scores than those couples who were assigned more routine nonchallenging tasks.

Novelty changes your brain chemicals and may help promote connection and intimacy. Explore and try new things—not only in the bedroom!

Novelty changes your brain chemicals and may help promote connection and intimacy. Explore and try new things—not only in the bedroom! Climb a mountain or dance in the living room—take a tap dancing or cooking course together. The concept is novelty. For those who are a bit skeptical, try something easy like breaking normal routine patterns. When you go to your favorite restaurant actually try a different kind of food, have sex at a different time of the day—if you're a night person, try in the morning or vice versa. Also, a novel sexual position can be both exciting and wonderful.

93. What types of behaviors increase dopamine?

You don't have to have your ankles and wrists bound (unless you want to) in order to increase brain chemicals that make you feel romantically exhilarated. Any novel behavior, such as going to unfamiliar restaurants, tasting new cultural cuisines, visiting a new art museum, or taking a crisp drive in the country may suffice to reignite "old sparks." A roller coaster ride is able to boost dopamine! Look for activities that promote fear, novelty, and excitement. For people who are more inclined toward adventure, Dr. Fisher notes that any "quasi-dangerous activity," including going to a scary movie, hiking in the woods, riding a roller coaster, kayaking, and skiing, will markedly escalate dopamine and norepinephrine.

Some couples may also benefit from the adventure holiday! Use your imagination, and try something new, exciting, and invigorating today!

94. What other brain chemicals are important for our sex life? What activities increase those?

Another pro-romance brain chemical is **oxytocin**. It is nicknamed the "cuddle hormone" because it is released primarily through skin-to-skin contact and is associated with feelings of security and attachment to a partner. The importance of touch for humans is not a new concept. In his book *Touching: The Human Significance of the Skin*, psychologist Ashley Montagu underscores the physical and mental importance of touching for humans. He points out that touch is associated with stress reduction, positive coping skills, a heightened sense of well-being,

Oxytocin

Hormone associated with milk ejection from the breast.

increased immunoglobin levels, pain reduction, and faster wound healing. So, how do you raise those oxytocin levels? Just a few minutes of stroking, hugging, cuddling, or massaging raises oxytocin in the body, as does nipple stimulation, genital stimulation, and orgasm.

95. Why do we seem to have more sexual energy and excitement when we are on vacation?

Think about the last time you were on a wonderful restful vacation. You may have laid on the same beach with the same book as last year, but chances are the beach (or the mountains or the European city) represented a break from the daily work and personal stress and monotony of your daily life and introduced some level of novelty, thus raising romantic brain chemicals.

Sometimes your brain needs a vacation from cancer as well. You have spent a lot of time and money focused on your treatment and rehabilitation. Certain things are constant reminders of the cancer experience. Some women even grow to dislike the color pink, as it reminds them of breast cancer. Physically getting some distance from the cancer can be helpful for the woman and her partner. Cancer was all-consuming and took up much time and effort—it is now time for a needed break for both your body and mind.

Endorphins

One of the body's own painkillers, an opioid (morphine-like) chemical produced by the body that serves to suppress pain.

In addition, while on vacation, most people are more physically active, increasing heart rates, blood flow to all parts of the body (including the genitals) and facilitating brain **endorphins** (feel-good chemicals) to release. Sometimes, on vacation, distractions like BlackBerries or cell phones are limited, and on occasion, adults even leave their children at home! Increased privacy can also help reignite your sexual life with your partner. Stress and fatigue, coupled with a nice feather bed and usually wonderful weather, can often set the stage for romance and rekindling of your sexual fire. Vacations revive, rejuvenate, and replenish our romantic stores, which easily become depleted with time, work, and family obligations.

These all combine to improve overall body image, positive outlook, and sexual self-esteem. Partners and women who have breast cancer should start planning their next vacation...right now!

96. How can we replicate these vacation feelings at home?

Many couples get stuck in a bit of a relationship "R.U.T." (routine, unimaginative, and tiresome). They come home exhausted after a long work week and look forward to a relaxing weekend watching the same television shows and barely interacting or conversing, much less making love.

Unfortunately, this type of "relaxation" does little to foster positive feelings within the relationship or to increase pro-sexual brain chemicals. To get out of this rut, plan weekly date nights. During these nights, television is prohibited, and novelty should be slowly introduced into everyday life. This need not be extravagant or expensive. You might start with a simple walk in the back yard or around the block. Then expand to visit an art gallery or a botanical garden. Each of the authors of this book has experienced the result of "letting life get too busy," and as such, we make concentrated efforts to incorporate some form of "date night" into our own relationships. We know that you will come to anticipate date nights and truly enjoy having dedicated, one-on-one couple time together. Try placing a note in his or her briefcase setting the stage. It's my turn tonight....I can't wait! An elusive text message may also build the anticipation.

97. What are "His and Hers" intimacy weekends?

His and Hers intimacy weekends are a very effective intimacy-enhancing technique. In his and hers weekends, one member of the couple takes responsibility for planning two novel and intimate experiences per month for the other. For instance, on the first and third weekends of the month, Mary is in charge of researching, planning, and executing intimate experiences for her partner, Tom. On the second and fourth weekends of the month, Tom reciprocates. "Intimate experiences" are not always sexual. Examples include going to a play that the partner would enjoy, trying a new restaurant, performing a back rub with scented oil, hiking on a mountainside, or having a rendezvous at a hotel. Couples agree to plan activities that will be welcome, not hurtful, to mind, body, or wallet. They are encouraged to "be good sports" and to participate in the activity that has been planned for them in the spirit of intimacy enhancement.

This challenges individuals to be as creative in date planning as they were when they first met. Intimacy experiences are often novel and fun and involve touch and hugging...raising all three pro-sexual brain chemicals!

98. What is fantasy play?

Fantasy play refers to the use of mental images or imaginary narratives that depart from reality. We all played dress up or had imaginary friends as children, but as adults, we often forget how to use fantasy to our sexual advantage. Research suggests that fantasies can arise spontaneously from the unconscious or be pursued consciously. This can be an important element of play and novelty introduction within a relationship and can drive creative thinking and artistic expression. Freud saw fantasy as a vehicle for the expression of desires.

Research suggests that fantasies can arise spontaneously from the unconscious or be pursued consciously.

Many women use fantasy play alone when they read erotic literature or view erotic films and then use images or scenarios from those mediums to augment their desire and arousal with their partner. This is a very common and healthy expression of sexuality. Other women incorporate fantasy into their sex play with a partner through activities such as dressing in costumes, acting out specific sexual scenarios, experimenting with bondage and submission role play, or re-enacting times from earlier in the relationship when the partner was a stranger that they were meeting for the first time. Any form of fantasy play that is safe and to which both members of a couple consent is perfectly normal and can provide a creative outlet for intimacy within a relationship.

Sharing sexual fantasies can be a great way to keep your relationship passionate and exciting. Rather than just telling your partner your own sexual fantasy, why not encourage him or her to do the same? Chances are you both have a sexual fantasy that you would like to share. This exercise of sharing your intimate thoughts and sexual desires can enhance the emotional and intimate connection you share with your partner. Focus on the communication aspects of sharing your thoughts. Try to be open and honest without passing judgment.

Create a Fantasy Suggestion Box. Each of you should write three to five intimate fantasies (they can be sexual but can also be a wild adventure together), and then put them in a suggestion box in the bedroom. Once a month, alternating, pull out a fantasy from the box and explore. By accepting and exploring each other's sexual fantasies, you will create an atmosphere of love, acceptance, and enhanced communication and will grow as individuals and as a couple.

99. What specific books can "spice things up"?

Enjoying erotic literature is a perfectly normal part of nourishing your sexual self. Your interest in a sexual enhancement through books and fantasy does *not* necessarily represent your desire for certain activities in your real life, but may be simply interesting and novel. After you purchase any of the books in the following list, commit to read for at least 20 minutes three times per week. Initially, during your reading, you should be alone and relaxed without demands or interruptions. Then you may wish to read aloud with your partner. Most selections can be found at your local library or favorite bookstore. Enjoy!

Instructional "Spicy" Reading
Becoming Orgasmic (by Heiman and LoPicolo)
The Elusive Orgasm (by Cass)

The Busy Couple's Guide to Great Sex (by McAllister and Rallie)

The Art of Kissing (by Cane)

The Big O (by Paget)

Lover's Weekend Guide (by Cooper)

Eat Chocolate Naked (by Johnson)

The Idiot's Guide to Amazing Sex (by Locker)

Sex for One/Orgasm for Two (by Dodson)

The Idiot's Guide to Tantric Sex (by Kuriansky)

Resurrecting Sex (by Schnarch)

The Good Girl's Guide to Bad Girl Sex (by Keesling)

Cancer and Sexuality (by the American Cancer Society)

Tantra for Erotic Empowerment (by Michaels and Johnson)

Discovering Your Couple Sexual Style: The Key to Sexual Satisfaction (by McCarthy)

Fictional Explicit "Spicy" Reading

The Best New Erotica (by Carroll and Groff)

Aqua Erotica (by Mohanraj)

The Blue Moon Erotic Reader (by Burner and Russet)

Erotic Interludes (by Barbach)

Forbidden Flowers or My Secret Garden (by Friday)

Erotic Edge or Pleasures (by Barbach)

Herotica (by Bright)

Erotic Fairy Tales (by Szereto)

Historical Erotica (by Carroll and Groff)

Dreamboat or The Parisian Affair (by Gould)

Bedtime Stories for Lovers (by Lloyd)

100. What specific resources can help us address sexual concerns and spice things up?

The Internet can be an immensely helpful adjunct for sexuality education and raising the romantic quotient. The following section lists helpful sites and other resources worth visiting.

Appendix: Resources

Websites

Hope Wellness Center
Founded by Sandra Finestone
www.HopeWellnessCenter.org

"Sex and A Healthier You"
A sexuality education program offered by The National Women's
Resource Center
www.SexandaHealthierYou.org

***uk*Cancer Back Up**
Information about the effect of cancer and cancer treatments on
sexuality.
www.cancerbackup.org.uk

The Center for Intimacy After Cancer Therapy Inc.
www.renewintimacy.org

The Society for Sex Therapy and Research (SSTAR)
Composed of highly skilled professionals who treat problems of sexual
function, sexual identity, reproductive life, and sexual issues related to
illness. Referral information is available from the SSTAR website.
www.sstarnet.org

For further information, please contact:
Society for Sex Therapy and Research
409 12th St., S.W., PO Box 96920
Washington, DC 20090-6920
202-863-2570

The North American Menopause Society
Educational material for the perimenopausal and postmenopausal woman.
www.menopause.org

The American College of Obstetricians and Gynecologists
Educational material an a number of women's health issues.
www.acog.org

WebMD Health and Sex Guide
www.webMD.com

National Vulvodynia Association and the International Pelvic Pain Society
Both sites have information about sexual pain, pelvic floor dysfunction and finding healthcare providers.
www.nva.org and *www.pelvicpain.org*

International Society for the Study of Women's Sexual Health
Information research on sexual health and finding a sexual medicine provider.
www.isswsh.org

American Association of Sex Educators, Counselors, and Therapists
Information about sexual health and finding a sex therapist, educator, or counselor.
www.aasect.org

Association of Reproductive Health Professionals
Information about sexual health.
www.arhp.org

Other Resources

American Cancer Society
1599 Clifton Road
Atlanta, GA 30329
1-800-ACS-2345
www.cancer.org

American College of Radiology
Preston White Drive
Reston, VA 20191-4326
703-648-8900
www.acr.org

American College of Plastic and Reconstruction Surgeons
444 East Algonquin Road
Arlington Heights, IL 60005
847-228-9900
www.plasticsurgery.org

American Society of Clinical Oncology
2318 Mill Road, Suite 800
Alexandria, VA 22314
571-483-1300
www.asco.org

Avon Breast Cancer Foundation
1345 Avenue of the Americas
New York, NY 10105
1-866-505-AVON
www.avoncrusade.com

BreastCancer.org
7 East Lancaster Avenue, Third Floor
Ardmore, PA 19003
www.breastcancer.org

Breast Cancer Network of Strength
135 South La Salle Street, Suite 2000
Chicago, IL 60603
1-800-221-2141
www.networkofstrength.org

Breast Cancer Network of Strength
Breast Cancer Network of Strength® provides immediate emotional relief to anyone affected by breast cancer through the YourShoes™ 24/7 Breast Cancer Support Center. YourShoes is the country's only 24-hour toll-free breast cancer hotline staffed exclusively by trained and certified peer counselors who are breast cancer survivors.

YourShoes peer counselors understand how important it is to talk with someone who's been through it themselves, and can help people touched by breast cancer feel the strength and support they need.

Our match program offers a chance for patients to be matched with peer counselors who have had similar diagnoses, treatment options, reconstruction choices, or life experiences—a woman or man who has walked in your shoes. Spouses and partners can also take advantage of our match program that supports people who are taking care of a wife or partner during breast cancer treatment.

Other services include a free wig and prosthesis bank for women with limited resources. Network of Strength Advocacy™ works to increase breast cancer research funding, support breast cancer related clinical studies, and ensure quality health care for all. *Networkofstrength.org* has message boards and more than 1,200 pages of easy to understand breast cancer content in seven languages.

Since breast cancer affects not just the patient but the whole family and circle of friends, anyone touched by breast cancer or who is concerned about breast health can use the Network of Strength's confidential and free services.

For more information about Breast Cancer Network of Strength, visit *www.networkofstrength.org*. Peer counselors can be e-mailed or contacted at 1-800-221-2141, with interpreters available in more than 150 languages.

Cancer Care, Inc.
275 Seventh Avenue
New York, NY 10001
1-800-813-HOPE
www.cancercare.org

Fertile Hope
1-888-994-HOPE
www.fertilehope.org

Gilda's Club Worldwide
48 Wall Street, 11th Floor
New York, NY 10005
1-888-GILDA-4-U
www.gildasclub.org

Her2 Support
6973 Mimosa Drive
Carlsbad, CA 92011-5156
www.her2supportgroup.org

Inflammatory Breast Cancer Research Foundation
321 High School Road
STE D##149
Bainbridge Island, WA 98110-2648
1-888-786-7422
www.ibcresearch.org

Lance Armstrong Foundation
2201 East Sixth Street
Austin, TX 78702
1-877-236-8820
www.livestrong.org

Living Beyond Breast Cancer
354 West Lancaster Avenue, Suite 224
Haverford, PA 19041
1-888-753-5222
www.lbbc.org

Mautner Project for Lesbians with Cancer
1875 Connecticut Avenue NW, Suite 710
Washington, DC 20009
1-866-628-8637
www.mautnerproject.org

Men Against Breast Cancer
Post Office Box 150
Adamstown, MD 21710-0150
1-866-547-MABC
www.menagainstbreastcancer.org

National Alliance of Breast Cancer Organizations
www.nabco.org

National Breast Cancer Coalition
1101 17th Street N.W., Suite 1300
Washington, DC 20036
1-800-622-2838
www.natlbcc.org

National Cancer Institute
31 Center Drive
Building 31, Room 10A31, MSC 2580
Bethesda, MD 20892-2580
1-800-4-CANCER
www.nci.nih.gov

NCI Clinical Trials
www.cancertrials.nci.nih.gov

NCI Genetics
www.cancer.gov/cancertopics/factsheet/risk/BRCA

National Center for Complementary and Alternative Medicine
Post Office Box 7923
Gaithenburg, MD 20898
1-888-644-6226
www.nccam.nih.gov

National Coalition for Cancer Survivorship
1010 Wayne Avenue, Suite 770
Silver Springs, MD 20910
1-888-650-9127
www.canceradvocacy.org

National Comprehensive Cancer Network
275 Commerce Drive, Suite 300
Fort Washington, PA 19034
1-888-909-NCCN
www.nccn.org

RESOURCES

National Lymphedema Network
1611 Telegraph Avenue, Suite 1111
Latham Square
Oakland, CA 94612-2138
1-800-541-3257
www.lymphnet.org

Oncology Nursing Society
125 Enterprise Drive
Pittsburgh, PA 15275-1214
1-866-257-4ONS
www.ons.org

Partnership for Prescription Assistance
1-888-477-2669
www.pparx.org

Patient Advocate Foundation
700 Thimble Shoals Blvd., Suite 200
Newport News, VA 23606
1-800-532-5274
www.patientadvocate.org

Susan G. Komen for the Cure
5005 LBJ Freeway, Suite 250
Dallas, TX 75244
1-800-GOKOMEN
www.komen.org

The Wellness Community
918 18th Street NW, Suite 54
Washington, DC 20006
1-888-793-WELL
www.wellness-community.org

Triple Negative Breast Cancer Foundation
Post Office Box 204
Norwood, NJ 07648
646-942-0242
www.tnbcfoundation.org

Young Survival Coalition
61 Broadway, Suite 2235
New York, NY 10006
1-877-YSC-1011
www.youngsurvival.org

Breast Cancer: Taking Control
Dr. John Boyages, an expert who has traveled the road of breast cancer with thousands of patients, takes you by the hand and guides you through the complex treatment maze.
www.breastcancertakingcontrol.com

RESOURCES

A

Acupuncture: A traditional Chinese practice of treating a health condition or medical state by inserting needles into the skin at specific points to unblock the flow of energy.

Alopecia: Loss of hair.

Antidepressant: The best medication to treat depression and panic attacks. They are nonaddictive and may benefit the central nervous system in many ways.

Aphrodisiac: A substance believed to improve or enhance sexual function or pleasure. Some think it may stimulate feelings of love, intimacy, or desire.

Areola: The circular patch of darker skin that surrounds the nipple. It is present in men and women.

Aromatase inhibitors: Drugs that suppress the body's natural production of estrogen by reducing production of the enzyme aromatase.

Aromatherapy: An integrative care practice that uses oils from plants to treat physical or psychological conditions. The oils can be inhaled, used in vaporizers, or used in massage.

Artherosclerosis: A condition in which fatty material collects along the walls of arteries.

Arthralgia: Joint muscle discomfort.

Axilla region: Armpit, underarm, or oxte.

B

Bilateral salpingo-oophorectomy: The surgical term for the removal of both the right and left fallopian tubes and ovaries.

Bioidentical hormones: Hormonal preparations, usually animal or plant derived, that have a similar structure to humans' naturally occurring hormones.

C

Cancer: A disease characterized by uncontrolled cell growth that ultimately causes destruction of normal healthy tissue.

Candida: Yeast infection typically occurs in the vagina and can be associated with itchiness and vaginal discharge.

Cardiovascular disease: The class of diseases that involve the heart or blood vessels (arteries and veins).

Chest wall radiation: Radiation to the chest.

Clitoris: The erectile organ in women whose external portion is located at the junction of the labia minora just in front of the vestibule.

D

Depression: A state of lowered mood usually associated with other disturbances like sleep, appetite, and loss of life's pleasure. Serious cases may be associated with suicidal thoughts.

Diabetes: A medical disease characterized with abnormal sugar metabolism and levels.

Dopamine: A catecholamine that serves as a neurotransmitter and also as a hormone inhibiting the release of prolactin from the anterior portion of the pituitary gland. It is involved in the neurochemistry of sexual function for both men and women.

Dyspareunia: Painful intercourse.

E

Endorphins: One of the body's own painkillers, an opioid (morphine-like) chemical produced by the body that serves to suppress pain.

Epithelial cell: Any one of several cells arranged in one or more layers that form part of a covering or lining of a body surface.

Erectile dysfunction: A persistent or recurrent inability to achieve or maintain an erection sufficient enough to accomplish a desired sexual behavior such as intercourse or coitus.

Erection: The expansion and hardening or stiffening of the sexual organ—it may be the penis, clitoris, or nipples—in response to sexual fantasy or stimulation.

Erotica: Sexually themed works such as books or sculpture deemed to have literary and artistic merit. Naked men, women, or other body parts are often featured as predominant themes.

Erythema: Redness following surgical procedure or local irritation.

Estradiol: The predominant sex hormone present in females.

Estrogen: A steroid hormone produced mainly in the ovaries; the primary female sexual hormone.

F

Female androgen insufficiency syndrome: A constellation of symptoms attributed to low testosterone levels in women. Some of the symptoms include fatigue, decreased well-being, a lack of energy or motivation, and decreased or absent sexual interest or desire.

Foreplay: Sexual behavior engaged in during the early part of the sexual encounter, with the aim of intensifying sexual arousal or pleasure.

Free radicals: An atom or group of atoms that has at least one unpaired electron and is therefore unstable and highly reactive. It typically can cause damage to normal cells.

G

G-spot: An area of increased erotic sensitivity on or deep inside the front of the vagina. It is located on the anterior surface of the vaginal vault. Stimulation in some women provides intense sexual pleasure.

H

High-density lipoproteins (HDL): A complex of lipids and proteins in approximately equal amounts that functions as a transporter of cholesterol within the bloodstream.

Hirsutism: Excessive hair growth.

Homophobia: Range of negative attitudes and feelings towards homosexuality and people identified as gay or lesbian.

Hormone therapy: The use of medications to modify or replace those whose production is decreased or absent in the menopause period.

Hypercholesterolemia: The presence of an abnormal amount of cholesterol in the cells and plasma of the blood.

Hypertension: High blood pressure; an abnormality in arterial blood pressure that typically results from a thickening of the blood vessel wall. It is a risk factor for many illnesses, including heart attacks, heart failure, and stroke, or end-stage kidney disease.

Hypoactive sexual desire disorder (HSSD): Lowered sexual interest that is often characterized by absence of sexual thoughts and fantasies—often associated with distress.

Hypersomnia: A sleep disorder characterized by excessive amounts of sleepiness.

Hysterectomy: Surgical removal of the uterus.

I

Insomnia: Disorder with sleep—inability to fall asleep.

Intercourse: Sexual contact usually involving coitus or penile vaginal penetration.

K

Kegel pelvic exercise: Exercise designed to increase muscle strength and elasticity in the pelvis. It may be recommended in the treatment of urinary incontinence.

L

Labia majora: Outer vaginal lips.

Labia minora: Inner vaginal lips.

Letrozole: An antiestrogen type of medication in the class of aromatase inhibitors. It inhibits the conversion of testosterone to estrogens.

Libido: Sexual interest or desire.

Lubrication: The natural appearance of slippery secretions in the vagina during sexual arousal or the use of artificial lubricants to facilitate sexual activity or intercourse.

Lumpectomy: Removal of a small amount of tissue of the breast including the abnormal cancerous cells.

M

Mammopexy: Breast lifting plastic surgical procedure.

Mammoplasty: Plastic surgery of the breasts; reduction—making breasts smaller; augmentation—making breasts larger.

Mastectomy: The removal of the breast.

Masturbation: The act of self-pleasuring; also known as self-stimulation.

Meditation: A complementary medicine practice of concentrated attention toward a single point of reference.

Medulla oblongata: An area of the brain.

Menopause: The lack of menstrual cycles for one year; the permanent end of a woman's menstrual cycle.

Mucosa: A surface layer of cells or epithelium that is lubricated by the secretions of mucosal glands.

N

Narcolepsy: A sleep disorder characterized by sudden and uncontrollable episodes of deep sleep.

Neuropathy: Damage to nerves of the peripheral nervous system.

Norepinephrine: A catecholamine with dual roles as a hormone and a neurotransmitter.

O

Oncoplastic surgery: Surgery in which a tumor is removed by either mastectomy or lumpectomy. Immediate reconstruction is performed at the time of surgery.

Orgasm: The intense pleasurable sensation at the peak of sexual activity or sexual climax usually associated with spasmodic contraction of the pelvic floor muscles.

Osteopenia: A condition characterized by bone loss.

Osteoporosis: A condition characterized by decrease in bone mass and density of the bones, resulting in "thinning" of the bones, causing them to become more fragile.

Ostomy: A bag that is on the outside of the body used to store fecal waste in the event of a urine, colonic, or anal resection.

Oxytocin: Hormone associated with milk ejection from the breast.

P

PDE5 inhibitor: Class of drugs which cause smooth muscle relaxation. Typically used in men and have been sued effectively for the treatment of erectile difficulties.

Penis: The erectile, sexually/erotically sensitive organ in males. The penis serves a sexual function and also mediates the voiding of urine.

Perineal area: The genital area between the vulva and anus.

Petechiae: Small hemorrhages.

Phosphodiesterase inhibitors: Drugs that block one or more of the five subtypes of the enzyme phosphodiesterase (PDE), therefore preventing the inactivation of the intracellular second messengers cyclic adenosine monophosphate (cAMP) and cyclic guanosine monophosphate (cGMP) by the respective PDE subtype(s).

Progesterone: A hormone that is secreted by the ovary and placenta (during pregnancy). It is necessary for pregnancy and has been implicated in female sexual function.

Progestin: A synthetic form of progesterone often used in birth control pills and hormone therapy.

Prophylactic mastectomy: Removal of the unaffected breast tissue.

Psychoanalytic therapy: A body of ideas developed by Austrian physician Sigmund Freud and continued by others. It is primarily devoted to the study of human psychological functioning and behavior, the primary focus is to reveal the unconscious content of a client's psyche in an effort to aleviate psychic tension.

R

Reactive desire: Desire that is triggered from an external stimuli rather than occuring spontaneously.

Reflexology: A therapeutic method of relieving pain by stimulating predefined pressure points on the feet and hands.

Reiki: A form of therapy that uses simple hands-on, no-touch, and visualization techniques, with the goal of improving the flow of life energy in a person.

Restless leg syndrome: A condition that is characterized by an irresistible urge to move one's body or legs to stop uncomfortable or odd sensations.

S

Scarguard: A series of topical skin-care products designed to be used together to minimize the appearance of scars from injury and surgery, and help prevent new scars from forming.

Selective serotonin reuptake inhibitor: A type of depressant medication that does not allow serotonin to be taken up again by the neuroreceptors, thereby causing more serotonin to be present in the neuron. These may be used for depression and panic attacks. Some include Prozac, Zoloft, Paxil, Celexa, Luvox, and Lexapro.

Sensate focus: A term used to describe a set of sexual exercises for couples or individuals. These exercises are aimed at increasing personal and interpersonal awareness of both our own and our partner's sexual needs.

Sexuality: The feelings, behaviors, and identities associated with sex.

Shiatsu massage: A manipulative therapy developed in Japan and incorporating techniques of anma (Japanese traditional massage), acupressure, stretching, and Western massage. Shiatsu involves applying pressure to special points or areas on the body in order to maintain physical and mental well being, treat disease, or alleviate discomfort.

Sildenafil: A phosphodiesterase inhibitor that is traditionally used in the treatment of male erectile dysfunction. New data support this class of medication that can sometimes be used for the treatment of SSRI-induced female sexual problems.

Sleep apnea: A sleep disorder characterized by pauses in breathing during sleep.

T

Tamoxifen: A selective estrogen receptor modulator that is used in the treatment of breast cancer.

Tantra: An ancient Indian spiritual tradition and belief system with the premise that sexuality is tied into personal energy and is capable of changing us if we submit to our primal sexual desires while maintaining control and heightening spiritual awareness. Tantra can intensify lovemaking and intensify the sexual dynamic or consciousness between couples.

Testosterone: A sexual hormone produced in the ovaries and adrenal glands. It is important in normal sexual functioning. It has been implicated in normal female libido or desire.

Thermography: Diagnostic technique using a thermograph to record the heat produced by different parts of the body; used to study blood flow and to detect tumors.

Trichomoniasis: A common sexually transmitted disease caused by the parasite Trichomonas vaginalis and infecting the urinary tract or vagina.

V

Vagina: The part of the female genital tract that connects the uterus to the external vulva. It is 8 to 10 cm in length.

Vaginal atrophy: When the vaginal tissues decrease in size and become pale or dry without lubrication, this is a result of decreased hormonal levels in the woman's body. The tissues can become sensitive, and often vaginal atrophy is associated with painful intercourse. This is commonly seen in chemical or natural menopause.

Vaginal dilators: Medical applications that can be placed within the vagina to help restore the vaginal tissues so that they are more adaptable.

Vaginal dyspareunia: Pain in the vaginal area during intercourse.

Vaginismus: An involuntary tightening of the vaginal muscles when the vagina is penetrated. The action can cause significant distress and pain.

Vaginitis: Inflammation of the vagina.

Vulva: The external genital organs of the female, including the labia majora, labia minora, clitoris, and vestibule of the vagina.

Y

Yoga: The spiritual practice aiming to unite the consciousness with universal consciousness to achieve harmony.

Yuan Chi: The genuine chi thought of as the life essence provided at conception by both parents.

GLOSSARY

A

INDEX

Other books in the *100 Questions & Answers* Series